Slow Cooker Recipes

The Tastiest Slow Cooker Recipes Around

Jessica Moore

Table of Contents

thought of as universal. As befitting its nature, it is presented without assurance regarding its prolonged validity or interim quality. Trademarks that are mentioned are done without written consent and can in no way be considered an endorsement from the trademark holder.

Introduction

Congratulations and thank you so much for purchasing *Slow Cooker Recipes*!

Many of us struggle with the hustle and bustle that inevitably comes to us every day. There is so much on your to-do list with never enough time to cross all of them off! While this book cannot help you organize your entire life, it can sure help you to become more efficient in the kitchen!

Pull the curtain back on an underrated kitchen appliance: the slow cooker! This baby takes the hard work out of cooking delicious, healthy meals for you and your entire family. All you have to do is mix, chop, and slice a few ingredients and dump them into your slow cooker! This magical and practical gadget does the rest. You can literally prepare a meal while you are away at work or doing busy doing things around your home. And that's not even mentioning the wonderful aromas that your slow cooker meals will bring you! Once you smell deliciousness, you know your meal is almost complete and ready to devour!

This cookbook is filled with a variety of easy to make recipes that are handpicked by a person, just like you, who wants the convenience of cooking at home but with a healthy spin! There are recipes for all occasions between these pages, waiting for you to discover and try them out for yourself!

While there are a plethora of slow cooker cookbooks, there is not one quite like this on the market! This book was written for the convenient but health-conscious at-home chefs. That being said, thank you so much for purchasing this book and adding it to your kitchen arsenal! Every effort was made to ensure it is full of as many valuable recipes as possible. Happy slow cooking!

Breakfast Recipes

Coconut Cream Pumpkin Quinoa Porridge

What's in it:

- 4 tbsp. honey
- ½ tsp. cinnamon
- 1/3 C. unsweetened shredded coconut
- 1/3 C. coconut cream
- 1 tbsp. coconut oil
- 1 – 1 ½ C. pumpkin puree
- 8 ounces water
- 12 ounces almond milk
- 1 ½ C. rinsed/uncooked quinoa

Optional Toppings:

- Coconut sugar
- Granola
- Gluten-free oats
- Nuts
- 2-3 tbsp. raw sugar
- Pinch of ginger

How it's made:

- Rinse quinoa and pour into slow cooker. Then add milk and set to warm for 30 minutes.
- Stir in pumpkin puree. Cook 8-10 more minutes until quinoa is fluffy.
- Add spices, coconut cream, and coconut oil, and combine well. Then add honey and shredded coconut.
- Spoon into serving bowls and top with toppings of choice or eat as is.

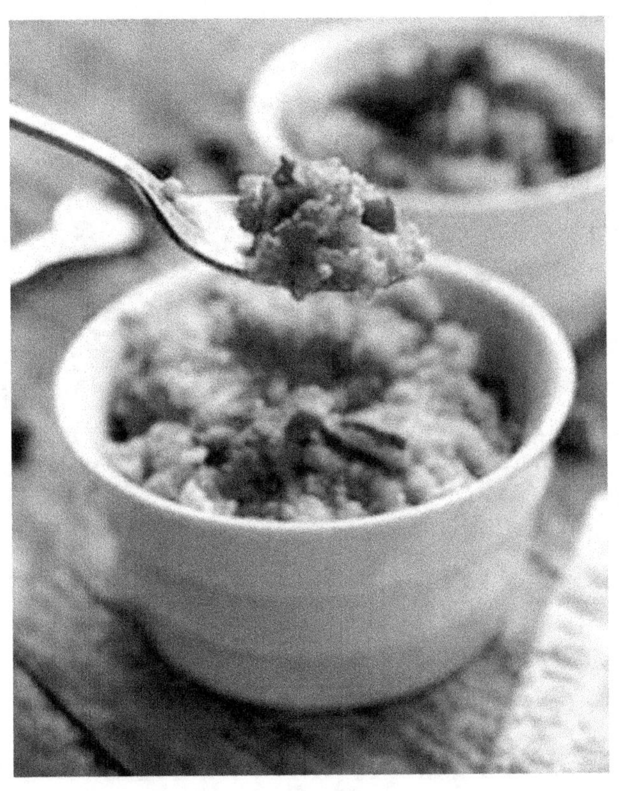

Breakfast Bake

What's in it:

- ½ tsp. pepper
- 1 tsp. salt
- 2 ½ C. almond milk
- 6 eggs
- 2 C. shredded sharp cheddar cheese
- 1 potato
- 2 C. cubed ham
- 3-4 C. broccoli florets
- 8-10 slices thick bread of choice

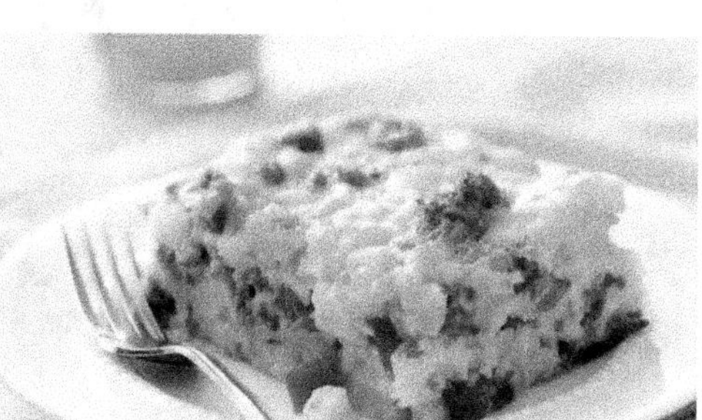

How it's made:

- Cut up ham and bread into cubes. Then shred cheese and potato.
- Layer the components into your slow cooker in this order: half of bread cubes, potato, half of cheese, half broccoli, ham, and remaining broccoli, cheese, and bread cubes.
- Mix milk, eggs, and seasonings and dump this mixture into the layers.
- Set to bake on low 6-7 hours. Eggs should be set and most of the liquid absorbed.

Apple Cinnamon Oatmeal

What's in it:

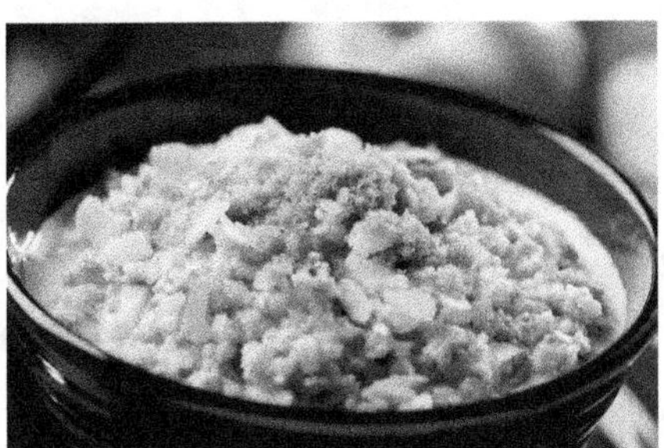

- ¼ tsp. salt
- 1 tsp. cinnamon
- 1 tsp. vanilla extract
- 1 tbsp. maple syrup
- 5 drops liquid stevia
- 1 C. chopped apple of choice
- 1 ½ C. unsweetened vanilla almond milk
- 2 ½ C. water
- 1 C. steel-cut oats

Serving Options:

- Dried fruit
- Coconut sugar
- Nut butter
- Chopped nuts

How it's made:

- Grease slow cooker with coconut oil.
- Pour in all recipe components into slow cooked and incorporate well.
- Set to slow cooker to low to cook 6-8 hours.
- Serve garnished with toppings of choice. Enjoy!

Gingerbread Oatmeal

What's in it:

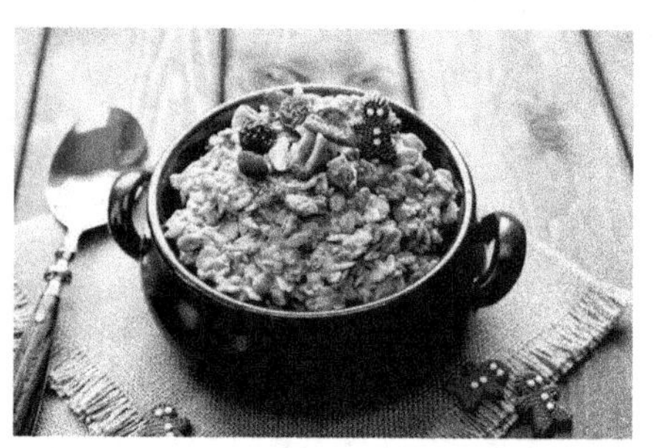

- 1 C. steel-cut oats
- ½ tsp. salt
- ¼ tsp. ground cloves
- 1 tsp. nutmeg
- 1 tsp. ginger
- 2 tsp. vanilla extract
- 1 tbsp. cinnamon
- 2 tbsp. dark brown sugar
- 2 tbsp. molasses
- 1 C. water
- 2 C. almond milk

How it's made:

- Grease slow cooker.
- Pour in all recipe components and combine well.
- Set to slow cooker to low to cook 8 hours.
- When ready to serve, fluff with a fork.
- Serve topped with a sprinkle of brown sugar, molasses, and chopped pecans if you desire.

Low-Carb Sausage and Egg Breakfast Casserole

What's in it:

- ¼ tsp. pepper
- ½ tsp. salt
- 2 minced cloves garlic
- ¾ C. whipping cream
- 10 eggs
- 1 C. shredded cheddar cheese
- 12 ounces cooked/sliced sausage links
- 1 head of broccoli

How it's made:

- Grease slow cooker.
- Cut up broccoli into florets and place half of broccoli into slow cooker. Then layer with only half of both sausage and cheese. The continue layering with remaining cheese, sausage, and broccoli.
- Whisk pepper, salt, garlic, whipping cream, and eggs together. Pour over layers.
- Set slow cooker to low to cook 4-5 hours or set to high to cook 2-3 hours till edges begin to brown.

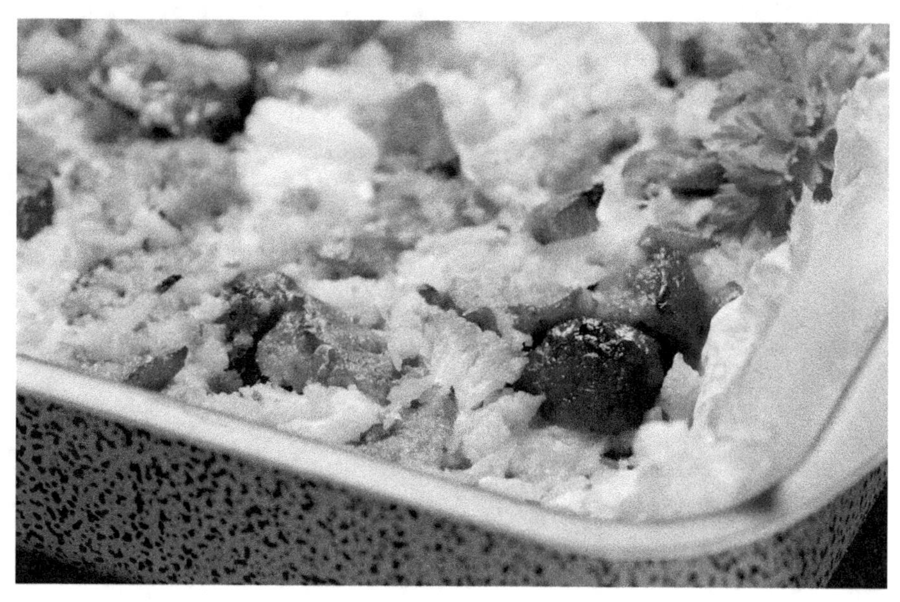

Chocolate Chip French Toast

What's in it:

- ¾ C. semi-sweet chocolate chips
- 1 tsp. cinnamon
- 1 tsp. vanilla extract
- ¾ C. brown sugar
- 1 ½ C. milk
- 3 eggs
- 1 loaf French bread

How it's made:

- Grease slow cooker.
- Cut French bread into cubes and place in an even layer in the bottom of slow cooker.
- Mix cinnamon, vanilla extract, sugar, milk, and eggs together. Pour over cubed bread. Toss to ensure even coating. Chill overnight.
- In the A.M., sprinkle with chocolate chips. and
- Set slow cooker to low to cook 4 hours. Enjoy!

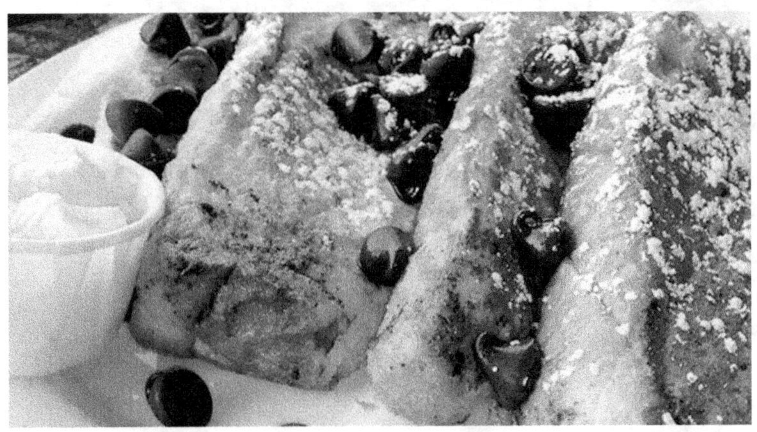

Coconut Cranberry Quinoa

What's in it:

- ¼ C. dried cranberries
- 1/8 C. sliced almonds
- 1/8 C. coconut flakes
- 3 tsp. honey
- 1 tsp. vanilla extract
- 1 C. uncooked quinoa
- 3 C. coconut water

How it's made:

- Pour all recipe components into your slow cooker.
- Set slow cooker to low to cook for 4 hours or Set slow cooker to high to cook 2 hours.

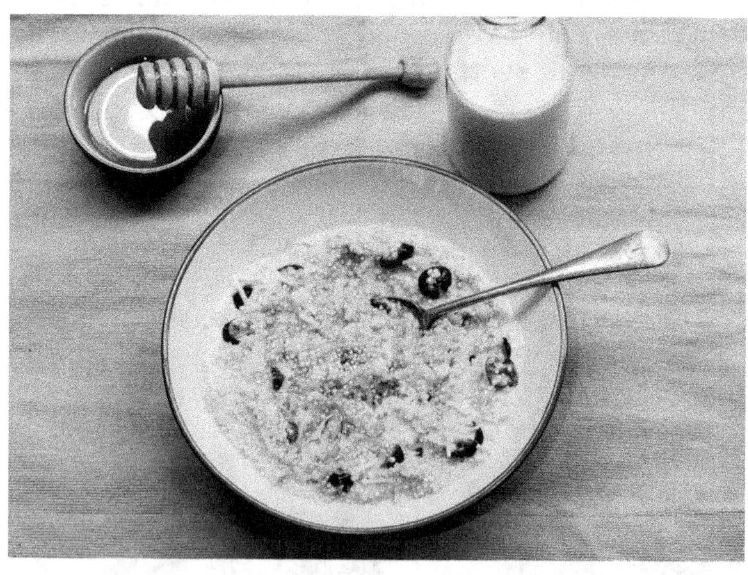

Veggie Omelet

What's in it:

- 1 minced clove garlic
- 1 chopped yellow onion
- 1 sliced red bell pepper
- 1 C. broccoli florets
- 1/8 tsp. chili powder
- 1/8 tsp. garlic powder
- Pepper
- ¼ tsp. salt
- ½ C. milk
- 6 eggs

Garnish:

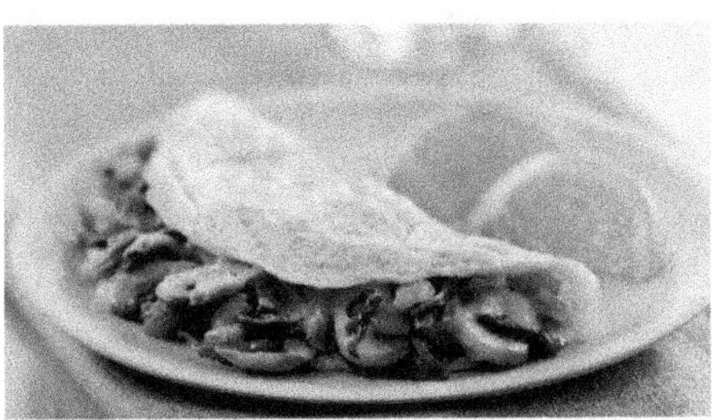

- Parsley
- Onions
- Tomatoes
- Shredded cheddar cheese

How it's made:

- Grease slow cooker.
- Combine chili powder, garlic powder, pepper, salt, milk, and eggs together.
- Place garlic, onions, peppers, and broccoli florets into the cooker. Pour egg mixture over veggies.
- Set slow cooker to high to cook 2 hours.
- Sprinkle with cheese and let sit 5 minutes till melted.
- Cut into wedges and serve topped with garnishes of choice.

Quinoa Energy Bars

What's in it:

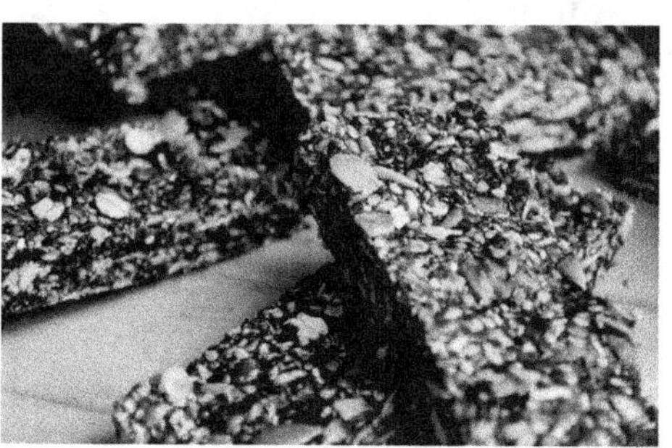

- 2 tbsp. chia seeds
- 1/3 C. chopped apples of choice
- 1/3 C. roasted/chopped almonds
- ½ C. raisins
- 1/3 C. uncooked quinoa
- 2 eggs
- ½ tsp. cinnamon
- Pinch of salt
- 1 C. unsweetened vanilla almond milk
- 2 tbsp. pure maple syrup
- 2 tbsp. almond butter

How it's made:

- Grease slow cooker. With parchment paper, cut a piece big enough to just sit at the bottom of cooker. Spray parchment paper.
- Combine maple syrup and almond butter. Then melt in microwave 30 seconds till creamy.
- Stir in salt and cinnamon into butter mixture. Then mix in eggs and remaining recipe components till well incorporated.
- Dump batter into your cooker. Set slow cooker to low to cook 3 ½ - 4 hours.
- When done, use a butter knife to run along edges. Chill till cooled.

- Cut into bars. A quick, on-the-go breakfast for you busy-bodies!

Pumpkin Chai Oats

What's in it:

- 1 cinnamon stick
- 2 tsp. vanilla extract
- 1 tbsp. chai spice
- 1 tbsp. pumpkin pie spice
- 1/3 C. brown sugar
- ¾ C. pumpkin puree
- 2 ½ C. unsweetened vanilla almond milk
- 2 ½ C. water
- 1 ½ C. steel cut oats

How it's made:

- Pour all recipe components into your slow cooker. Stir to incorporate.
- Set slow cooker to high to cook 2 hours.
- Remove cinnamon stick and stir well before devouring!

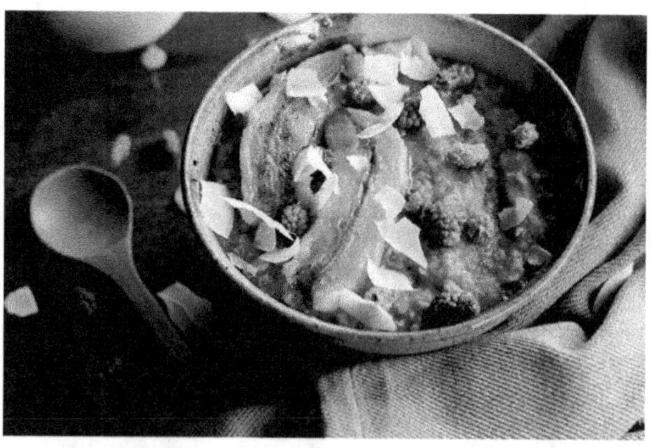

Lunch Recipes

White Bean Chicken Chili

What's in it:

- Pepper and salt
- 2 tsp. cumin
- Chili powder
- 4 diced zucchini
- 1 diced green bell pepper
- 1 diced onion
- 14.5-ounce can low-sodium chicken broth
- 3 16-ounce can great northern beans
- 4-ounce can fire roasted green chilies
- 1 pound boneless, skinless raw chicken breast

How it's made:

- Sauté garlic, zucchini, green pepper, and onions until translucent in color.
- Pour all recipe components into the slow cooker along with sautéed veggies.
- Set slow cooker to high to cook 4-5 hours or set slow cooker to low to cook 6-8 hours.
- Remove chicken from cooker and with forks, shred meat.
- Serve! (I like mine with a dollop of plain Greek yogurt for extra creaminess!)

Beef and Broccoli

What's in it:

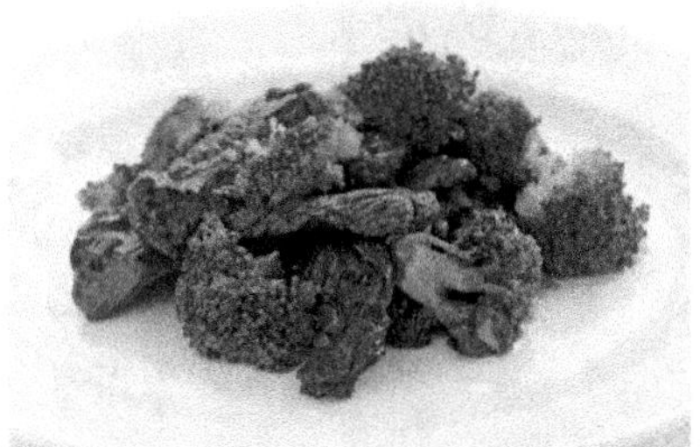

- 1 tbsp. canola oil
- 2 tbsp. cornstarch
- 5 minced cloves garlic
- ½ C. beef stock
- 3 C. broccoli florets
- 1 pound flank steak

Sauce:

- 2 tsp. cornstarch
- ¼ C. brown sugar
- ½ C. low-sodium soy sauce

How it's made:

- Slice beef and toss with cornstarch.
- Pour all recipe and sauce components into slow cooker.
- Set slow cooker to low to cook 6 hours.
- Toss everything well before serving.

Pineapple BBQ Meat Balls

What's in it:

- ½ C. brown sugar
- 20 ounces pineapple chunks in juice
- 18 ounces BBQ sauce of choice
- ½ bag frozen meatballs

How it's made:

- Pour meatballs into slow cooker.
- Then pour brown sugar, pineapple chunks and juice, and BBQ sauce over meatballs. Toss to ensure even coating.
- Set slow cooker to high to cook 1 hour. Once 60 minutes is up, turn down cooker to low and cook 2-3 more hours.

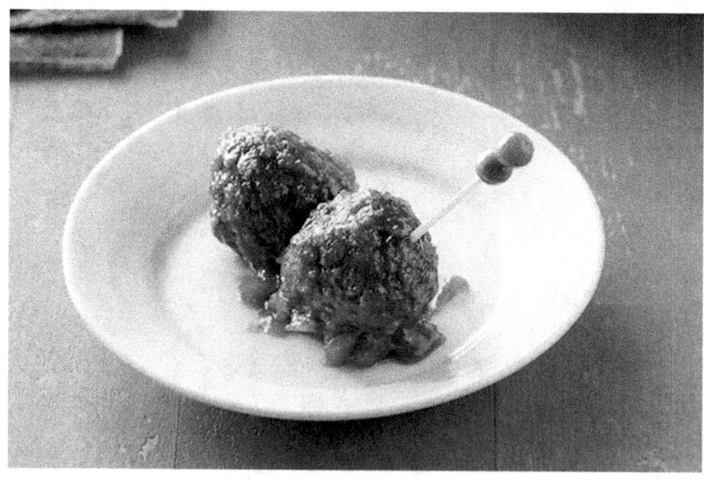

Chicken Pot Pie

- 1 bag frozen mixed veggies
- 1 can buttermilk biscuits
- ¼ tsp. pepper
- ¼ tsp. poultry seasoning
- ¼ tsp. celery seeds
- 2 cans cream of mushroom soup
- 1 diced white onion
- ¾ C. sliced celery
- 4 boneless, skinless chicken breasts

How it's made:

- Grease slow cooker. Cut up chicken into 1-inch cubes. Place chicken in the cooker, and top it with onion and celery.
- Pour pepper, poultry seasoning, and celery salt into the cooker. Then add cream of mushroom soup over veggies.
- Set slow cooker to low to cook 4 hours till chicken is completely cooked.
- As veggies cook, bake biscuits 13-15 minutes at 350 degrees.
- When serving, spoon chicken mixture onto a plate and top with a biscuit that is cut in half. Enjoy!

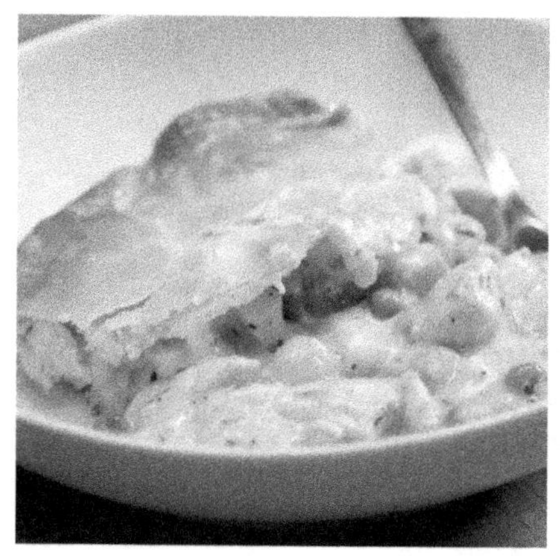

Pulled BBQ Chicken

What's in it:

- 18 ounces BBQ sauce of choice
- ½ tsp. pepper
- 1 tsp. salt
- 1 tsp. onion powder
- 1 tsp. garlic powder
- 2 pounds boneless, skinless chicken breasts

How it's made:

- Grease slow cooker.
- Put chicken into slow cooker, along with pepper, salt, onion, and garlic.
- Pour BBQ sauce over meat.
- Set slow cooker to high to cook 3-4 hours or set slow cooker to low to cook 6-7 hours.
- Take out chicken and shred. Put back into the cooker and warm everything through. Eat on sandwich buns.

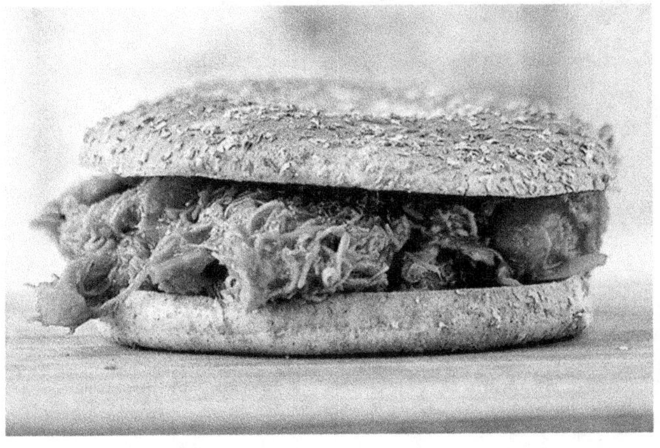

Chicken and Gravy

What's in it:

- Pepper
- 2 C. water
- 1 can low-fat, low-sodium cream of chicken soup
- 2 packages chicken gravy mix
- 6 boneless, skinless chicken breasts

How it's made:

- Grease slow cooker. Place chicken in cooker.
- Mix pepper, water, soup, and gravy mix together till well combined. Dump mixture onto chicken, making sure it covers meat thoroughly.
- Set slow cooker to LOW to cook for 4 hours till chicken is cooked.
- Serve with toast, brown rice, or mashed potatoes.

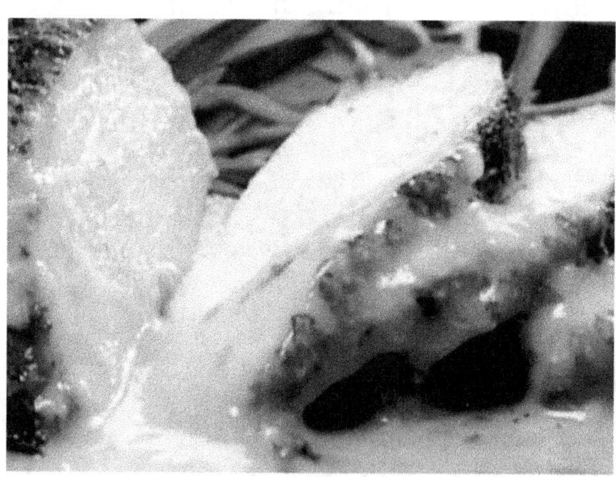

Pumpkin Chili

What's in it:

- ¼ tsp. pepper
- 1 tsp. salt
- 1 ½ tsp. cumin
- 1 tsp. cinnamon
- 2 tbsp. chili powder
- 2 ½ tsp. oregano
- ½ - 1 C. chicken broth
- 14 ounce can pumpkin puree
- 28-ounce can diced tomatoes
- 1 ½ pounds grass-fed bison or beef
- 6 minced cloves garlic
- 1 diced green bell pepper
- 2 C. chopped yellow onion
- 1 tbsp. coconut oil

How it's made:

- Sauté peppers and onions together 7 minutes till softened. Then add garlic and sauté 30 more seconds.
- Mix ground beef into mixture and brown 8-10 minutes till almost cooker.
- Pour meat mixture into slow cooker and add remaining recipe components.
- Set slow cooker to low to cook 6-7 hours.

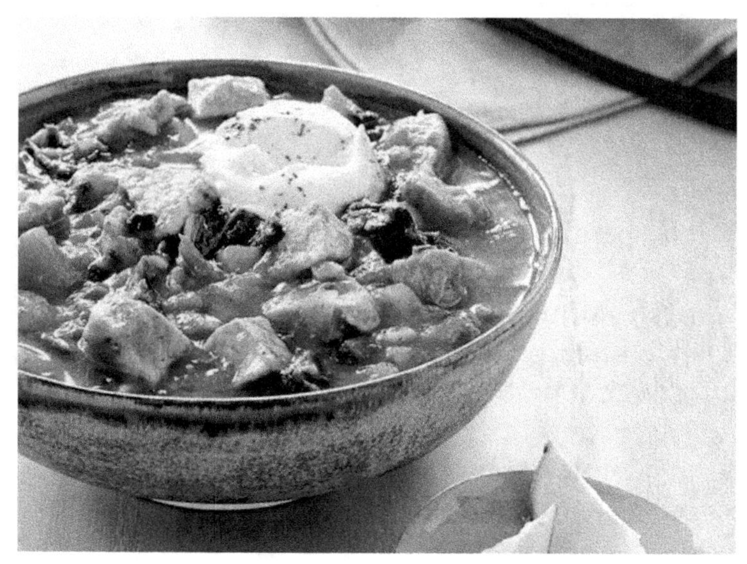

Mexican Shredded Beef

What's in it:

- 1 C. beef broth
- ½ C. Picante salsa
- 1 tsp. Mexican oregano
- 1 tsp. cumin
- 6 diced garlic cloves
- 1 C. diced onion
- 2 tbsp. tomato paste
- 1 tbsp. olive oil
- 1 ½ tsp. salt
- 1 tbsp. chili powder
- 3-4 pounds chuck roast

How it's made:

- Cut roast up into 2-inch cubes. Combine with chili powder and salt, tossing to ensure even coating. Brown meat in a pan.
- Place meat in slow cooker. Set slow cooker to low to cook 6-7 hours or Set slow cooker to high to cook 4-5 hours.
- Serve on top of tortillas with a lime wedge and a drizzle of lime juice.

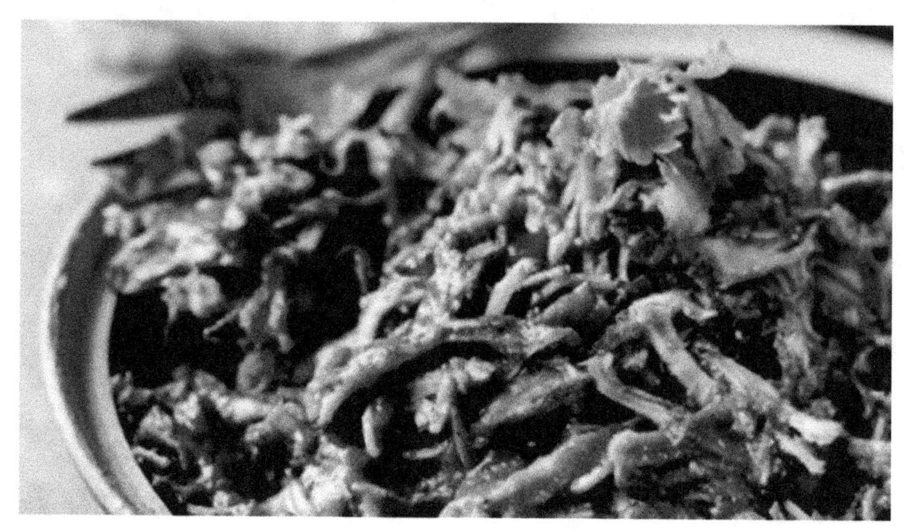

Parmesan Pork

What's in it:

- ¼ C. cold water
- 2 tbsp. cornstarch
- ½ tsp. salt
- 2 tbsp. olive oil
- 2 tbsp. minced garlic
- 2 tbsp. Italian seasoning
- 3 tbsp. soy sauce
- 1 tbsp. basil
- ½ C. honey
- 2/3 C. grated parmesan cheese
- 1 pound boneless while pork loin roast

How it's made:

- Slice roast in half and put into slow cooker.
- Combine salt, oil, garlic, basil, soy sauce, honey, and cheese together. Dump over meat, making sure it covers meat thoroughly.
- Set slow cooker to low to cook 5-6 hours till pork is thoroughly cooked through.
- Take out meat, covering with foil to keep warm.
- Strain fat from cooking liquids and pour into small pan. Bring mixture to boiling.
- Mix cold water and cornstarch together and add to boiling cooking liquid.
- Slowly stir in cornstarch mixture. Bring to boil and stir 2 minutes till the mixture becomes thick.
- Drizzle sauce over pork when serving. Enjoy!

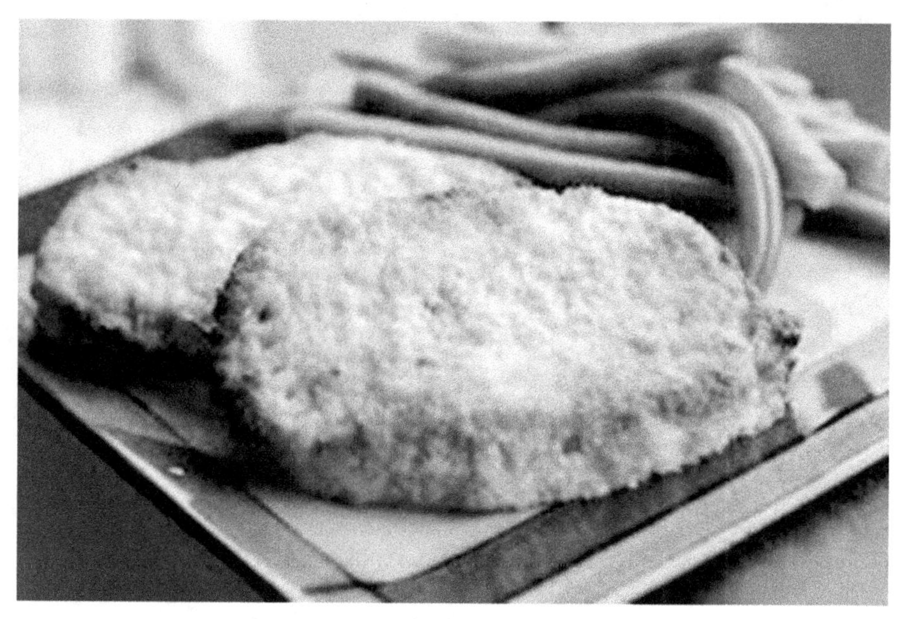

Italian Red Wine Roast Beef

What's in it:

- ¼ tsp. pepper
- 1 tsp. salt
- ½ tsp. marjoram
- ½ tsp. thyme
- 1 tsp. basil
- ½ C. red wine
- ½ C. water
- 1 sliced onion
- 2 ½ pounds beef round roast

How it's made:

- Mix all spices together. Set to the side.
- Put roast into slow cooker and sprinkle spice mixture over meat. Top roast with onions and pour red wine and water into cooker.
- Set slow cooker to low to cook 8-10 hours. Meat will fall apart.
- Shred meat and toss with cooking juices.

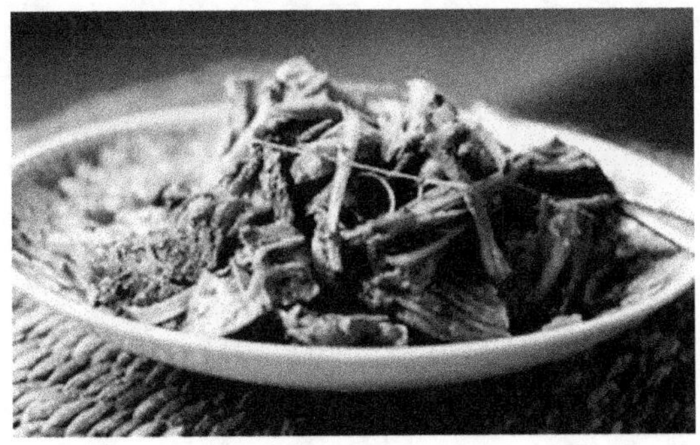

Snack and Appetizer Recipes

Crunchy Granola

What's in it:

- 1 C. dried fruit of choice
- ½ C. honey
- ½ C. melted coconut oil
- ¼ tsp. salt
- 2 C. shredded coconut
- 2 C. chopped nuts
- 4 C. old-fashioned oats

How it's made:

- Grease slow cooker liberally.
- Pour salt, coconut, nuts, and oats in the slow cooker.
- Melt coconut oil and mix in honey. Stir well and pour over contents in cooker.
- Set slow cooker to high to cook 30 minutes. You will want to stir every 20-30 minutes for about 2 – 2 ½ hours.
- When done, pour granola onto a sheet with a rim, spreading out in an even layer to cool.

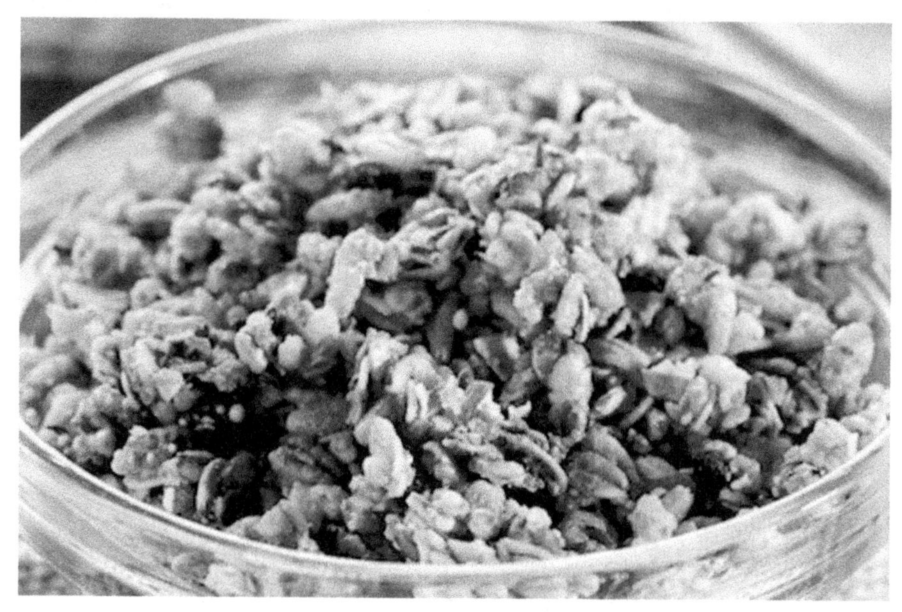

Boiled Peanuts

What's in it:

- 1/3 C. salt
- 2 quarts water
- 2 pounds green peanuts

How it's made:

- Pour peanuts into a colander and wash well under cold water. Then place into slow cooker. Cover with water, add salt and stir well.
- Set slow cooker to high to cook 5-6 hours.

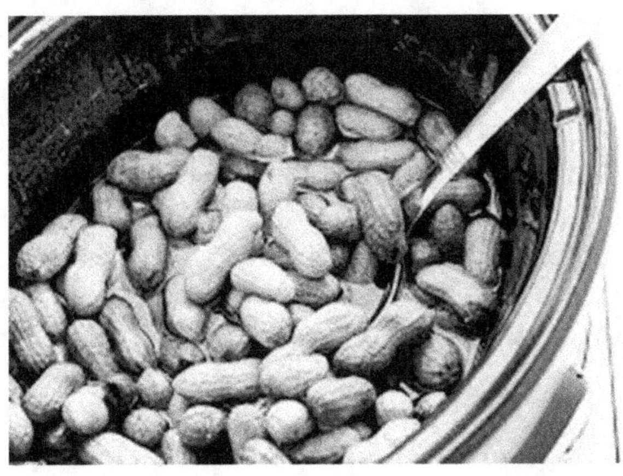

Cinnamon Apples

What's in it:

- 2 tbsp. unsalted butter
- Pinch of salt
- 3 tbsp. cornstarch
- 1/8 tsp. nutmeg
- 1 tbsp. cinnamon
- ½ C. brown sugar
- ½ C. granulated sweetener of choice
- 6 Granny Smith apples

How it's made:

- Peel and slice apples into thin pieces. Place into the slow cooker along with salt, cornstarch, nutmeg, cinnamon, brown sugar, and sweetener.
- Cube butter and mix into slow cooker.
- Set slow cooker to low to cook 4 hours or Set slow cooker to high to cook 2 hours. Make sure to stir 1-2 times during cooking process.
  Serve warm with whipped cream, ice cream, or as is!

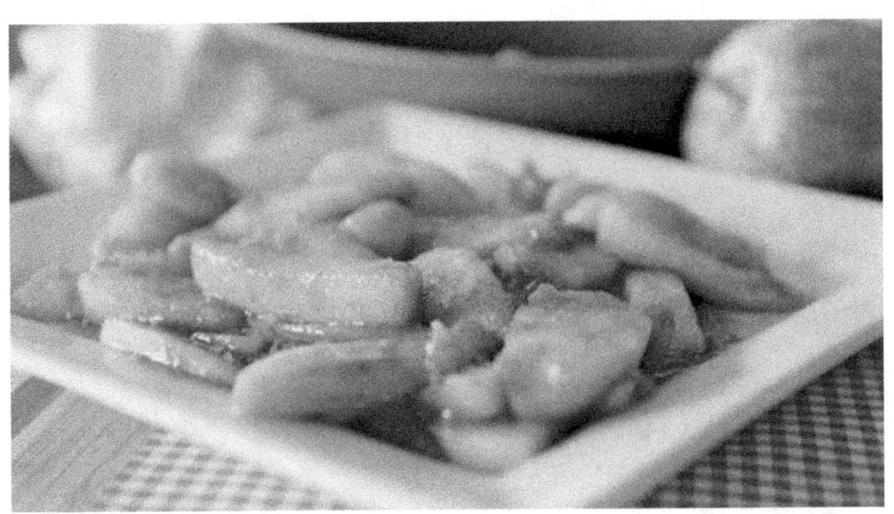

Pumpkin Spice Granola

What's in it:

- ¼ C. pumpkin seeds
- ½ C. pecan seeds
- 3 C. old-fashioned oatmeal
- ¼ tsp. salt
- 1 tbsp. pumpkin pie spice
- ¼ C. pumpkin puree
- 2 tsp. vanilla extract
- ¼ C. honey
- 2 beaten egg whites

How it's made:

- Mix salt, pumpkin pie spice, pumpkin puree, vanilla extract, honey, and egg whites together.
- Place pumpkin seeds, oatmeal, and pecans into the slow cooker and cover with honey mixture. Fold till well incorporated.
- Set slow cooker to high to cook 2-3 hours. Ensure you crack the lid to allow moisture to escape and prevent granola from getting soggy.
- Transfer cooked granola on a sheet to cool.

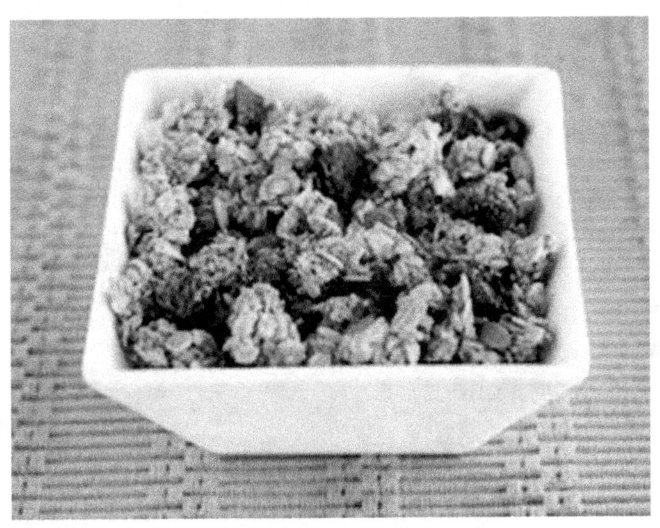

Spicy Chili Con Queso Dip

What's in it:

- ½ tsp. salt
- Dash of Worcestershire sauce
- 4-ounces can chopped green chili peppers
- 4 ounces shredded cheddar cheese
- 3 ounces cream cheese
- ¾ C. salsa of choice
- ¼ C. chopped onion
- 1 tbsp. butter

How it's made:

- Add all recipe components to a slow cooker. Combine well.
- Set slow cooker to low to cook 3 hours.
- Serve with favorite chips, crackers, etc.

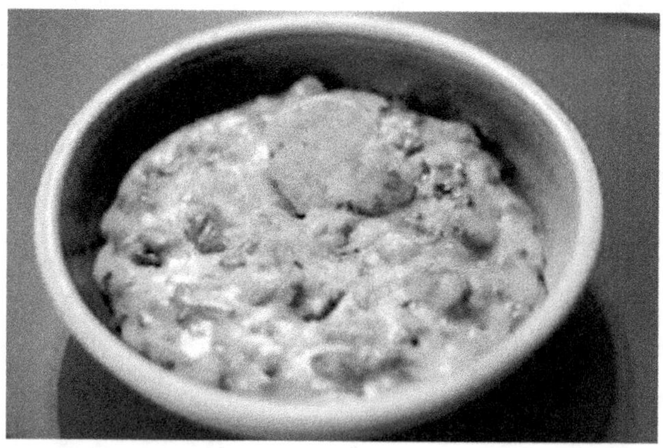

BBQ Chicken Meatballs

What's in it:

- 1 C. BBQ sauce of choice
- 1/8 tsp. cayenne pepper
- 1/8 tsp. allspice
- 1/8 tsp. nutmeg
- ¼ tsp. pepper
- ½ tsp. salt
- ½ tsp. rubbed sage
- ½ tsp. thyme
- ½ tsp. minced garlic
- ¼ C. chopped onion
- 3 tbsp. milk
- 2 slices torn bread
- 1 pound boneless, skinless chicken thighs

How it's made:

- Trim fat off chicken and cut into chunks.
- Soak bread in milk for 5 minutes.
- Combine seasonings, onion, chicken pieces, and soaked bread in a food processor. Mix till blended.
- Pour mixture into slow cooker. Set slow cooker to high to cook 2 hours till cooked through.
- Heat BBQ sauce and pour over cooked meatballs and enjoy!

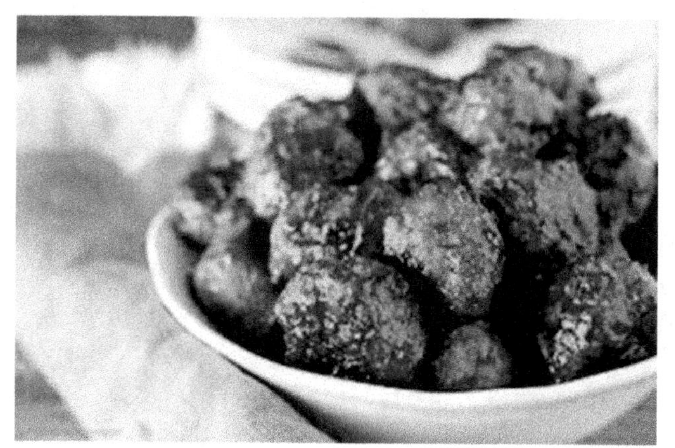

Cajun Spiced Pecans

What's in it:

- ¼ tsp. cayenne pepper
- ¼ tsp. garlic powder
- ½ tsp. onion powder
- 1 tsp. thyme
- 1 tsp. oregano
- 1 tsp. basil
- 1 tsp. salt
- 1 tbsp. chili powder
- ¼ C. melted butter
- 1 pound pecan halves

How it's made:

- Pour all recipe components into your slow cooker.
- Set slow cooker to high to cook 15 minutes.
- Then turn cooker to low, uncover and cook 2 hours, stirring on occasion.
- Place mixture on a sheet and allow to cool.

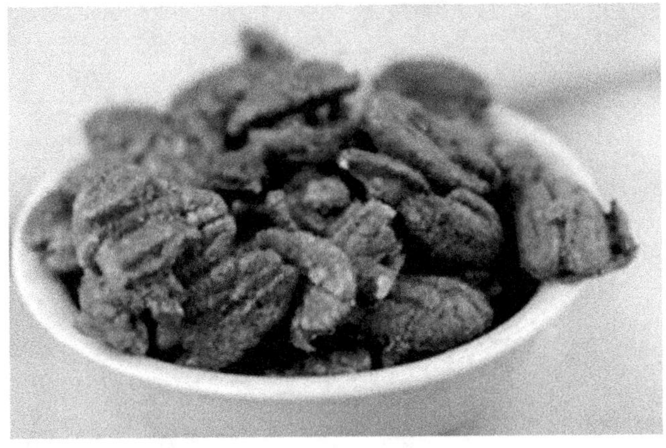

3-Ingredient Cheese Salsa Dip

What's in it:

- 16-ounce jar salsa of choice
- 16 ounces cubed Velveeta cheese
- ½ C. chopped cilantro

How it's made:

- Place salsa and cheese into slow cooker. Set slow cooker to high to cook 2 hours.
- Stir in cilantro.
- Serve with corn or tortilla chips. Enjoy!

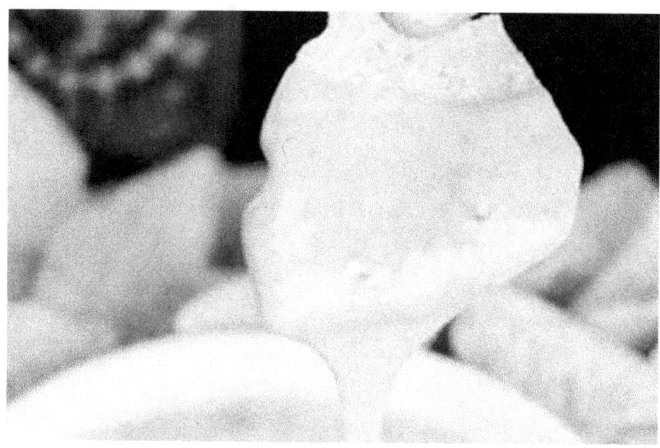

Chili Cheese Taco Dip

What's in it:

- 1 pound Mexican shredded cheese
- 1 can chili with no beans
- 1 pound ground beef

How it's made:

- Brown beef and drain grease. Add to slow cooker.
- Add cheese and chili to slow cooker. Set slow cooker to low to cook 1 – 1 ½ hours till ingredients are well blended, and cheese is melted.
- Serve warm!

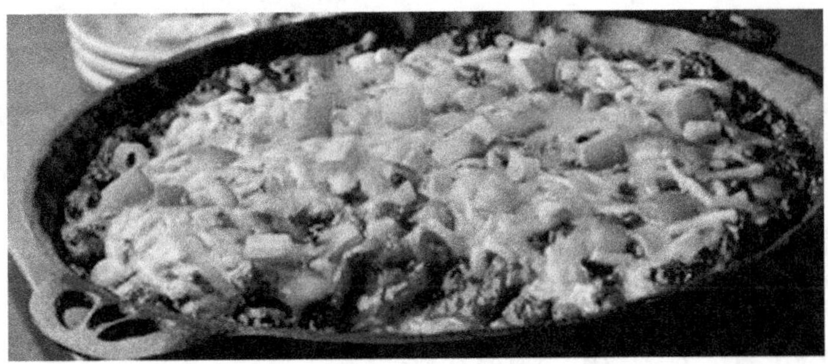

Teriyaki Chicken Wings

What's in it:

- 2 minced cloves garlic
- 2 tbsp. ginger
- 1 tbsp. chili garlic paste
- ¼ C. dry sherry
- 1 C. brown sugar
- 1 C. low-sodium soy sauce
- 1 chopped onion
- Pepper and salt
- 3 pounds chicken wings

How it's made:

- Rinse chicken wings and pat dry. Chop off wing tips and cut each at the joint to create two sections.
- Sprinkle wings with pepper and salt. Broil wings 8-10 minutes per side.
- Mix garlic, ginger, chili paste, sherry, brown sugar, soy sauce, and onion together.
- Place broiled wings into the slow cooker and pour garlic mixture over meat.
- Set slow cooker to low to cook 4 hours or set slow cooker to high to cook 1 ½ - 2 ½ hours.

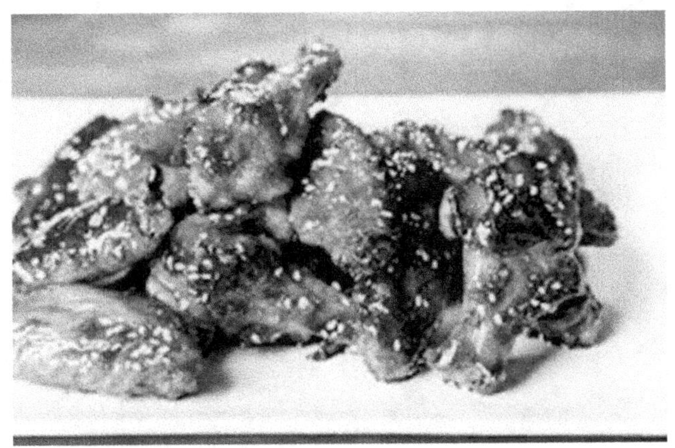

Side Recipes

Mexican Quinoa and Rice

What's in it:

- 3 minced cloves garlic
- ¼ C. tomato paste
- 2 ½ C. vegetable broth
- 1 tsp. chili powder
- 1 tsp. salt
- 1 tbsp. olive oil
- 1 C. rinsed quinoa
- 1 C. quick cooking brown rice

How it's made:

- Grease slow cooker and add chili powder, salt, olive oil, quinoa, and rice. Combine well.
- Warm vegetable broth to a simmer in a pan. Stir in tomato paste and garlic. Then pour over quinoa mixture.
- Set slow cooker to low to cook 2 hours.
  When done the cooking, remove the lid and put a clean towel over the cooker. Put the lid back on and allow mixture to sit 10 minutes before serving.

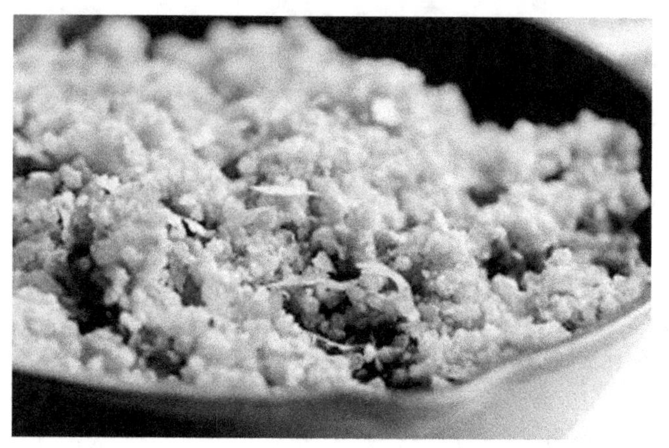

Southern Green Beans

What's in it:

- 1 ½ pounds trimmed green beans
- ¼ tsp. salt
- 1 C. chicken broth
- 1 chopped onion
- 3 slices bacon

How it's made:

- Cook bacon until crispy. Reserve 1 tsp of bacon grease.
- Sauté onion in bacon grease 5 minutes until tenderized.
  Crumble cooked bacon and set to the side.
- Combine green beans, onion, salt, and chicken broth in your slow cooker.
- Set slow cooker to low to cook 8 hours till beans become tender.
- Pour beans onto a serving platter. Top with crumbled bacon.

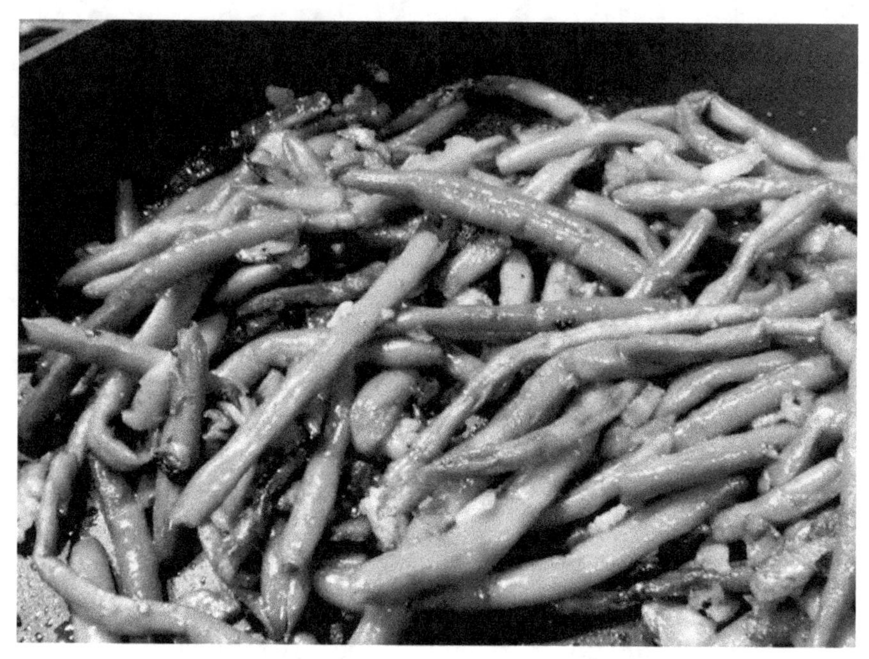

Loaded Mashed Cauliflower

What's in it:

- 1 tsp. steak spice
- 1 chopped green onion
- 3 pieces bacon
- ½ C. shredded cheddar cheese
- ½ C. sour cream
- 1 C. water
- 2 tsp. rosemary
- 3 tsp. minced garlic
- 1 head cauliflower

How it's made:

- Slice head of cauliflower into florets and pour into slow cooker.
- Add water, steak spice, garlic, and rosemary to cooker.
- Set slow cooker to low to cook 5-6 hours till cauliflower becomes soft.
- Drain water. Add the majority of sour cream, cheese, bacon and green onion.
- Mash cauliflower mixture till you achieve the consistency you desire.
- Serve garnished with leftover sour cream, bacon bits, shredded cheese and green onion.

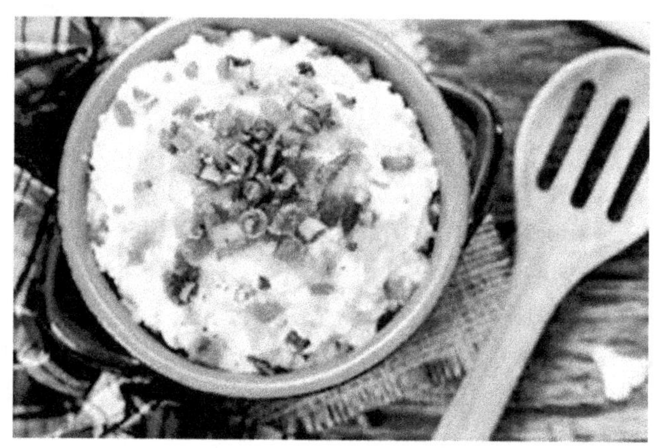

Garlic Parmesan Spaghetti Squash

What's in it:

- Pepper and salt
- ½ C. grated parmesan
- ¼ C. heavy cream
- 3 minced cloves garlic
- 6 tbsp. unsalted butter
- 1 spaghetti squash

How it's made:

- With a sharp knife, pierce spaghetti squash 10 times around the entire squash. Place in slow cooker. Set slow cooker to high to cook 3-4 hours or on low 6-8 hours.
- When squash is tender, take out of slow cooker and let cool a bit. Slice lengthwise and remove seeds.
- Scrape flesh with a fork, creating long strands.
- Place flesh back into slow cooker and turn it to low. Add butter, garlic, and cream, stirring well. Cook on low until creamy and thickened.
- Pour in parmesan cheese and stir. Season with pepper and salt as needed
- Serve with parsley leaves as a garnish. Enjoy!

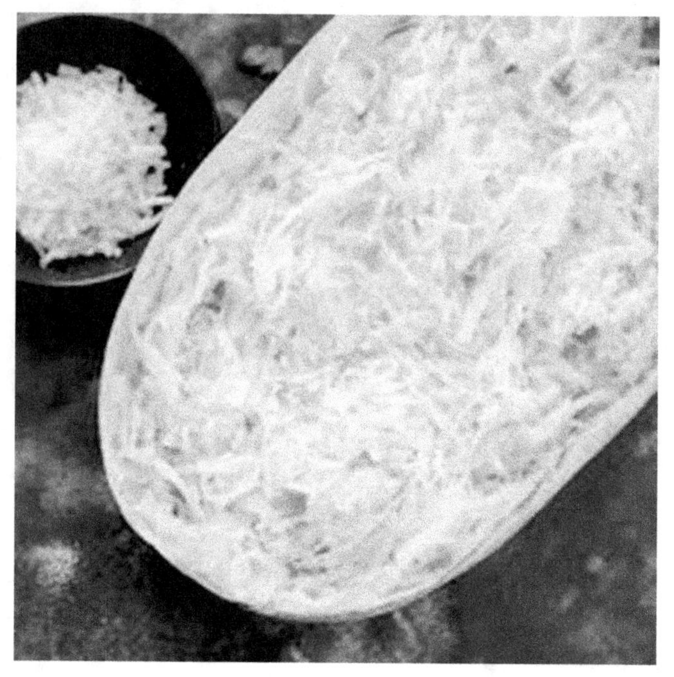

Garlic Parmesan Potatoes

What's in it:

- ¼ C. parmesan + more for serving
- 1 tsp. oregano
- 1 tsp. thyme
- ¼ tsp. pepper
- ¼ tsp. salt
- 3 minced garlic cloves
- ¼ C. olive oil
- 3 pounds small red potatoes

How it's made:

- Wash and cut potatoes into wedges and place into slow cooker.
- Mix oregano, thyme, pepper, salt, garlic, and olive oil together. Pour over potatoes and gently toss to coat. Sprinkle with parmesan cheese.
- Set slow cooker to high to cook 3 hours.
- When serving, top with additional parmesan cheese.

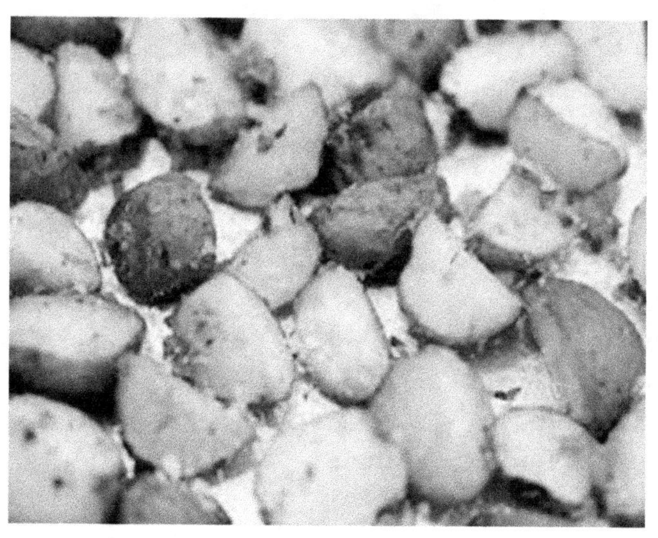

Slow Cooker Dinner Rolls

What's in it:

- Melted butter
- 3 – 3 ½ C. flour
- ¾ tbsp. salt
- ¾ tbsp. yeast
- 1 ½ C. warm water

How it's made:

- Mix water, salt, and yeast together. Then add flour and combine well to create a dough.
- Cover dough and allow time to double in size.
- Punch dough and chill till ready to use.
- With parchment paper, line your slow cooker and grease paper and inside of cooker.
  Split up dough into 8 sections and form into balls. Place into the cooker.
- Set slow cooker to high to cook 1 hour.
- Once no longer sticky, they are done!
- Brush with melted butter and broil until crust becomes crisp.

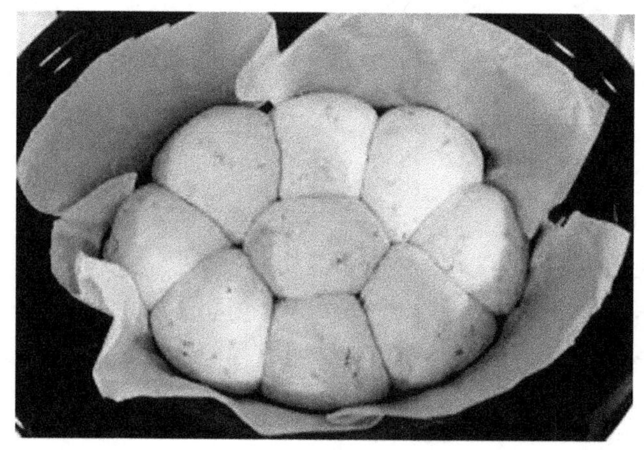

Cheesy Mushroom Quinoa

What's in it:

- 1 C. shredded parmesan cheese
- Pepper and salt
- 1 tsp. Italian seasoning
- 1 tbsp. minced garlic
- 4 ounces cream cheese
- 8 ounces sliced mushrooms
- ½ diced red bell pepper
- 2 chopped green onions
- 2 C. uncooked quinoa
- 4 C. vegetable broth

How it's made:

- Place all recipe components into slow cooker minus cheese.
- Set slow cooker to high to cook 2-3 hours or Set slow cooker to low to cook 4-5 hours.
- Mix all components together. Sprinkle cheese on top and let sit 15 minutes to melt.

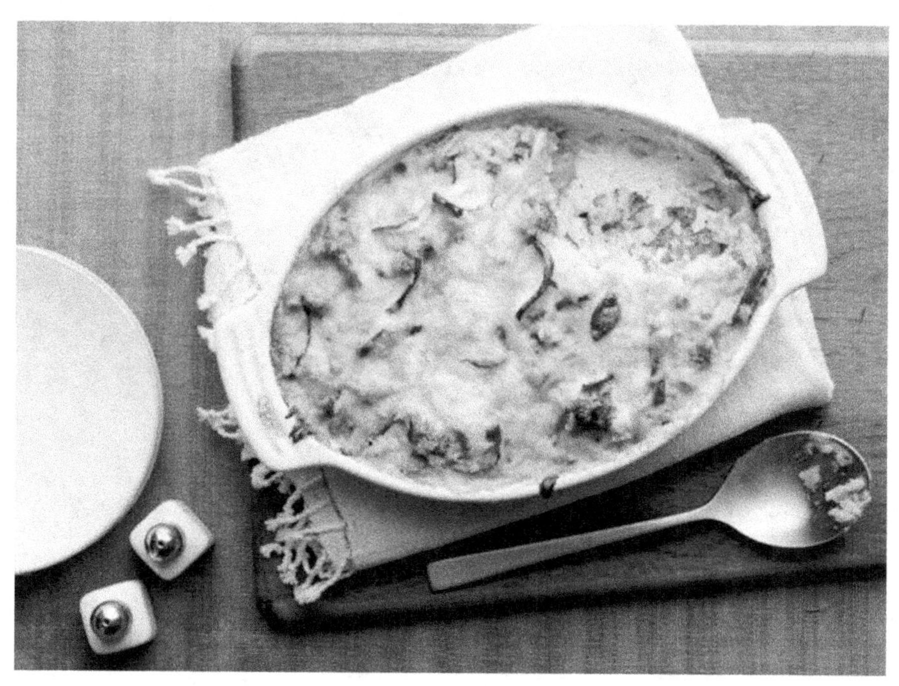

Cheesy Broccoli Rice

What's in it:

- 1 ¼ C. cheddar cheese
- 2 C. chopped broccoli
- 1/3 tsp. pepper
- 1 ¼ tsp. salt
- 32 ounces chicken broth
- 1 C. uncooked long grain rice
- 1 chopped garlic cloves
- 1 chopped onion
- 1 tbsp. olive oil

How it's made:

- Put garlic, onion, and olive oil into slow cooker. Add rice, pepper, and salt and combine well.
- Pour 2/3 of chicken broth in. Set slow cooker to high to cook 4 hours.
- Add broccoli and stir. Add more broth if needed.
- Cook 30 more minutes till broccoli becomes tender and bright green in color.
- Add cheese and stir until melted. Season with pepper and salt to achieve desired taste.

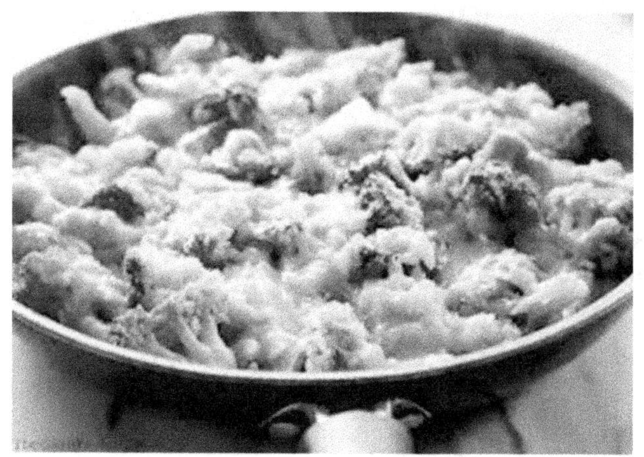

Brown Sugar Carrots

What's in it:

- ½ tsp. salt
- ½ tsp. cinnamon
- ½ C. brown sugar
- ¼ C. unsalted butter
- 5 pounds carrots

How it's made:

- Place all recipe components into slow cooker.
- Set slow cooker to low to cook 4 hours.
- Serve sprinkled with a bit more brown sugar.

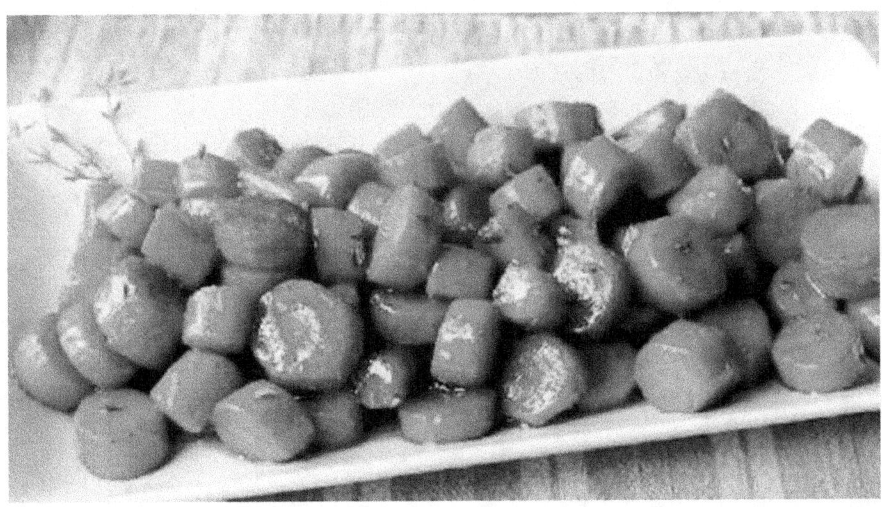

Mashed Sweet Potatoes

What's in it:

- Pinch of cinnamon
- Pinch of nutmeg
- Pinch of salt and pepper
- 1-2 tbsp. ghee
- ¾ C. water
- 2-3 pounds sweet potatoes

How it's made:

- Wash, peel, and slice sweet potatoes into chunks. Place in the slow cooker along with pepper, salt, and water.
- With parchment paper, cover sweet potatoes. Cover and Set slow cooker to high to cook 2-3 hours till potatoes become tenderized.
- With a potato masher, mash until creamy. Stir in ghee and serve warm!

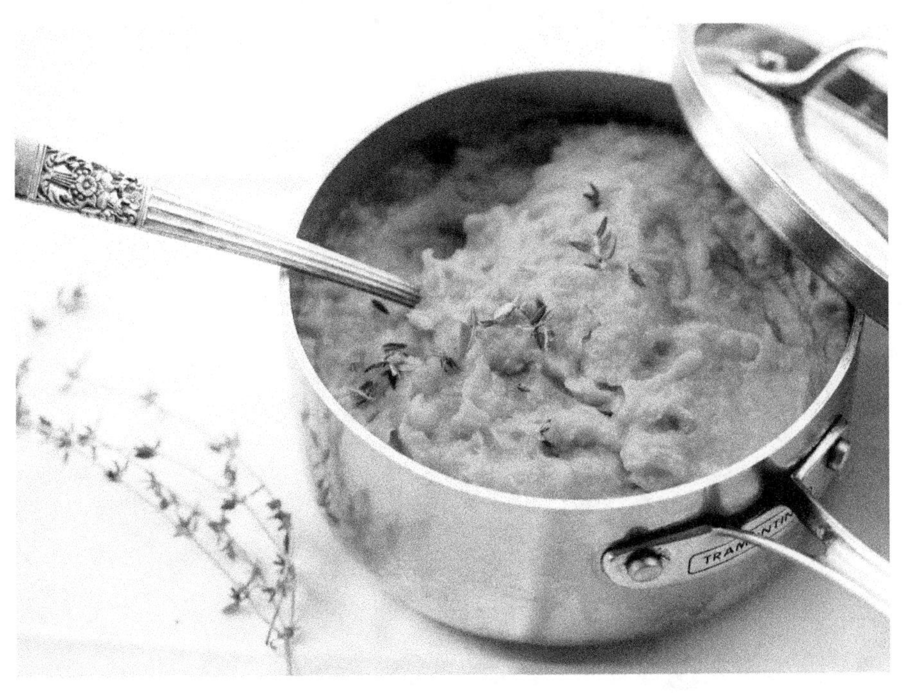

Soup and Stew Recipes

Buffalo Chicken Soup

What's in it:

- ¼ C. chopped green onions
- ¼ C. crumbled blue cheese
- ½ C. tortilla chip strips
- 4 C. chicken stock
- ¼ C. blue cheese dressing
- ¼ C. hot cayenne sauce
- 1 pound boneless skinless chicken breast
- 3 sliced celery stalks
- 3 sliced carrots
- 2 minced cloves garlic
- ½ peeled/chopped onion
- 1 tbsp. butter

How it's made:

- Melt butter in a skillet and sauté celery, carrots, garlic, and onion together until soft.
- Pour sautéed veggies into the slow cooker along with chicken stock, blue cheese dressing, cayenne sauce, and chicken breast.
- Set slow cooker to high to cook 2-3 hours or set slow cooker to low to cook 4-5 hours.
- Remove chicken and shred. Place back into the cooker.
- Serve topped with tortilla strips, green onions, and crumbled blue cheese.

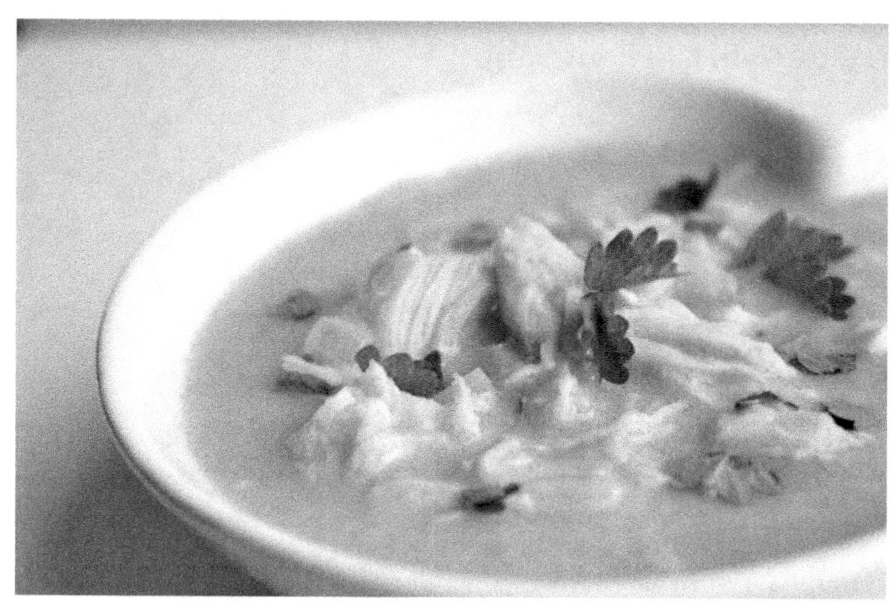

Sweet Potato, Chicken, and Quinoa Soup

What's in it:

- 5 C. chicken broth
- 1 packet chili seasoning mix
- 1 tsp. minced garlic
- 14.25 ounce can petite diced tomatoes
- 15.25 ounce can black beans
- 2 pounds sweet potatoes
- 1 C. quinoa
- 1 ½ pounds boneless skinless chicken breasts

How it's made:

- Grease slow cooker.
  Trim fat from chicken breasts and place into the slow cooker along with rinsed quinoa.
- Remove skins from potatoes and chop into chunks and pour them into the cooker.
- Drain/rinse black beans and place into cooker along with chicken broth and can of tomatoes.
- Set slow cooker to high to cook 3-5 hours.
- Shred chicken with forks and mix mixture well to incorporate all ingredients.
- Season with pepper and salt if needed and garnish with parsley.

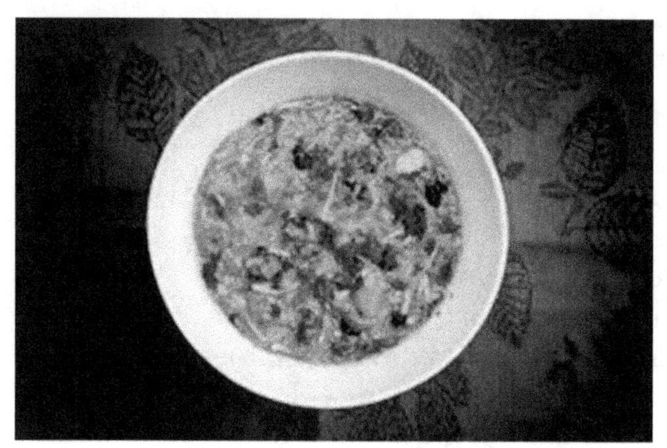

Chicken Korma with Sweet Potato

What's in it:

- 2 sweet potatoes
- 8 boneless skinless chicken thighs
- 14 ounce can coconut milk
- 2 crushed cloves garlic
- 1 tsp. sugar
- 2 sliced onion
- 2 tbsp. olive oil
- 4 tsp. water
- 1 tsp. salt
- 1 tsp. paprika
- 1 tsp. chili powder
- ½ tsp. turmeric
- 3 tsp. cumin
- 3 tsp. coriander

For serving:

- 2 tbsp. ground almonds
- 1 tbsp. lemon juice
- 2 tsp. garam masala

How it's made:

- Combine all spices together, mixing in just enough water to create a paste from spice mixture. Set to the side.
- Warm oil and sauté sugar and onions together till light gold. Then add garlic and cook 60 seconds. Mix in spice mixture and cook 2 minutes till toasted.

- In a blender, mix coconut milk with spice-garlic-onion mixture, blending until smooth. Pour into slow cooker.
- Place sweet potatoes and chicken into the cooker, tossing to evenly coat.
- Set slow cooker to low to cook 3-4 hours.
- To serve, mix in serving ingredients. Serve with rice and/or naan bread.

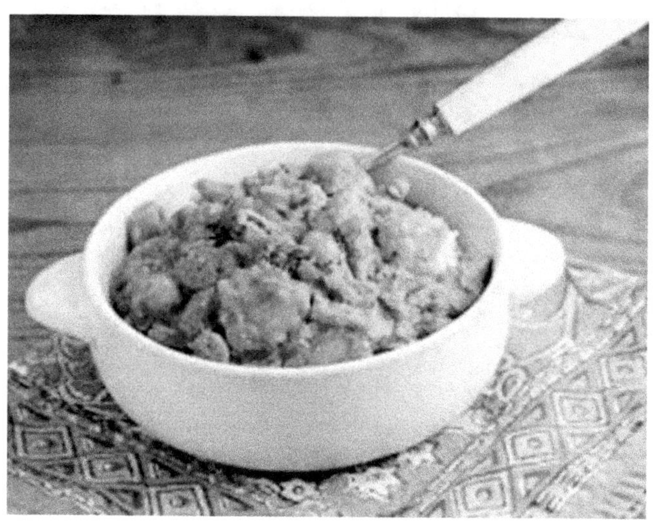

Chicken Potato Soup

What's in it:

- Pepper and salt
- 1/3 C. chopped parsley
- 1 tsp. thyme
- 8 C. chicken broth
- 2 C. sliced celery
- 2 C. sliced carrots
- 1 ½ pounds boneless skinless chicken breast
- 3 pounds russet potatoes
- 3 minced cloves garlic
- 1 peeled/chopped onion
- 4 chopped slices bacon

How it's made:

- Cook bacon and add garlic and onion. Sauté 3-4 minutes. Pour mixture into slow cooker.
- Put chicken on top of garlic mixture. Then add ½ tsp pepper, 1 ½ tsp. salt, broth, celery, carrots, and potatoes.
- Set the slow cooker to high to cook 8-12 hours.
- Take out the chicken and stir soup well to break up potatoes.
- If you want a creamy soup, use an immersion blender to blend soup contents.
- Serve with cheese and parsley.

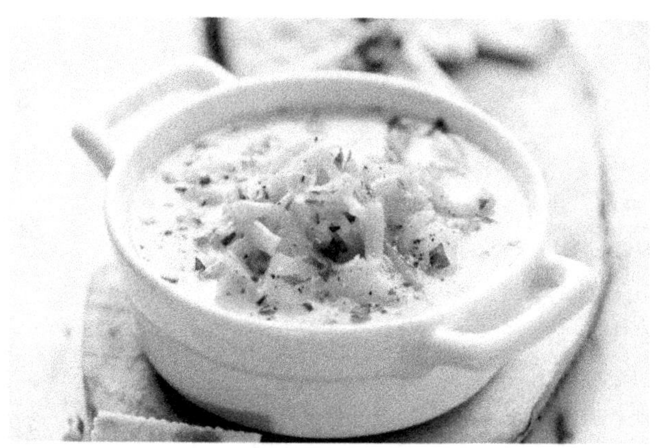

Broccoli and Cheese Soup

What's in it:

- 8 ounces grated sharp cheddar cheese
- ¼ tsp. pepper
- ½ tsp. salt
- 12 ounce can evaporated milk
- 2 ½ C. low-sodium chicken broth
- ¼ tsp. nutmeg
- 1 tsp. oregano
- 2 ounces cream cheese
- 3 minced cloves garlic
- 1 diced yellow onion
- 1 C. grated carrots
- 5 C. chopped broccoli florets

How it's made:

- Put garlic, onion, carrots, and broccoli into slow cooker. Then add broth, nutmeg, oregano, and cream cheese. Stir to combine.
- Set slow cooker to high to cook 2 hours or Set slow cooker to low to cook 4-6 hours till broccoli becomes tender.
- Mix in evaporated milk.
- Puree ¾ of soup with an immersion blender.
- Warm soup on low for 10-15 minutes to warm through.
- Season with pepper and salt and add grated cheese.

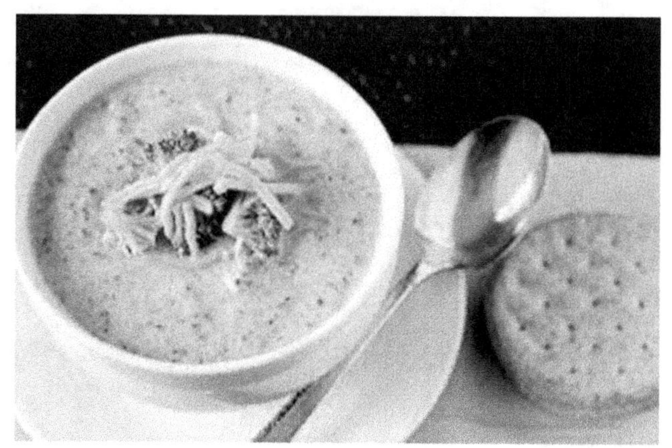

Sausage, Spinach, and White Bean Soup

What's in it:

- 3 C. baby spinach leaves
- Pepper and salt
- 4 C. chicken broth
- 2 bay leaves
- ½ tsp. oregano
- 2 15-ounce cans great northern beans
- 2 diced stalks celery
- 3 diced carrots
- 1 diced onion
- 3 minced cloves of garlic
- 1 package andouille sausage
- 1 tbsp. olive oil

How it's made:

- Warm up olive oil. Thinly slice sausage and add to pan, cooking 3-4 minutes till just browned.
- Pour bay leaves, oregano, beans, celery, carrots, onions, garlic, and sausage into slow cooker. Mix in 2 cups of water along with chicken broth. Season with pepper and salt.
- Set slow cooker to low to cook 7-8 hours or Set slow cooker to high to cook 3-4 hours.
- Stir in spinach till it becomes wilted.

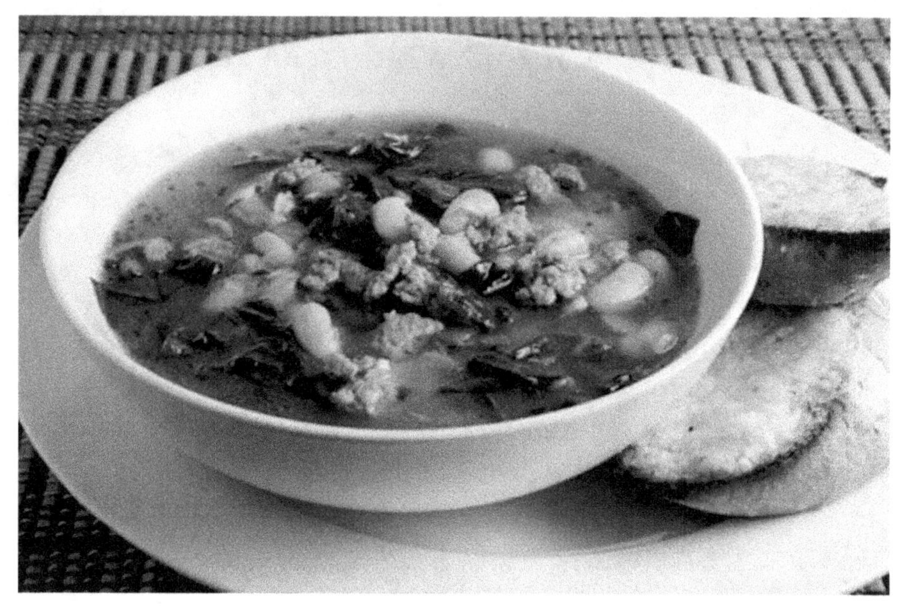

Harvest Beef Stew

What's in it:

- Pepper and salt
- 2 tbsp. minced parsley
- 1 tsp. Italian seasoning
- 1 tbsp. balsamic vinegar
- 4 C. water
- 28 ounce can diced tomatoes
- 4 minced cloves garlic
- 1 chopped onion
- 3 C. russet potatoes
- 3 diced celery ribs
- 2 C. sliced carrots
- 3 tbsp. olive oil
- 1/3 C. whole wheat flour
- 1 beef chuck roast

How it's made:

- Cut roast into ½-inch chunks. Diced potatoes into ½-inch chunks.
- Mix flour with beef cubes. Sauté beef 5-10 minutes till browned. Place into slow cooker.
- Place seasonings, vinegar, water, tomatoes, garlic, onion, potatoes, celery, and carrots to meat in slow cooker. Incorporate well.
- Set slow cooker to low to cook 5-6 hours. Season with pepper and salt as needed.

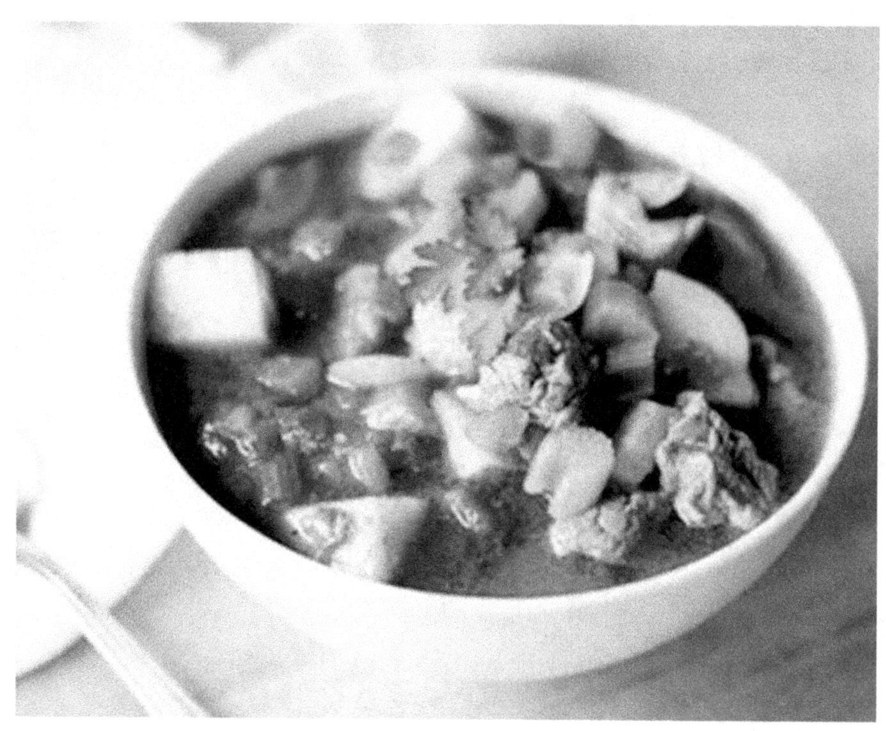

Black Bean Soup

What's in it:

- ½ tsp. cayenne pepper
- 2 tsp. salt
- 2 tsp. chili powder
- 2 tsp. cumin
- 4 15-ounce cans black beans
- 4 C. vegetable stock
- 1-2 jalapeno peppers
- 5 minced cloves garlic
- 2 chopped carrots
- 2 chopped red bell peppers
- 1 chopped onion

Optional Toppings:

- Shredded cheese
- Sour cream
- Avocados
- Crumbled tortilla chips
- Cilantro

How it's made:

- Drain black beans, chop, and de-seed jalapeno peppers.
- Mix all ingredients in your slow cooker.
- Set slow cooker to low to cook 6-8 hours or Set slow cooker to high to cook 3-4 hours till veggies are tenderized.
- You can serve as is or pour into a food processor to blend till you reach desired consistency.

- Top with desired toppings when serving.

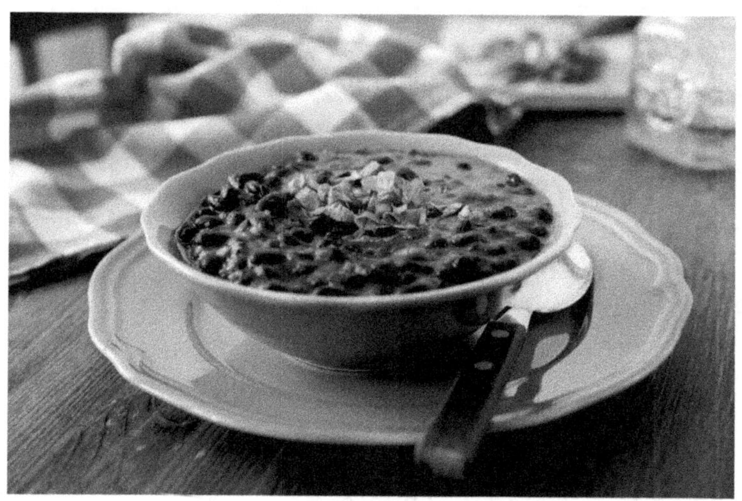

Spiced Carrot and Lentil Soup

What's in it:

- 1 C. milk
- ½ C. vegetable stock
- ¾ C. split red lentils
- 4 C. washed/chopped carrot s
- 2 tbsp. olive oil
- Pinch of chili flakes
- 2 tsp. cumin seeds

How it's made:

- Dump all recipe components into your slow cooker.
- Set slow cooker to low to cook 5 hours till carrots become softened.
- With an immersion blender, blend soup until creamy and smooth.

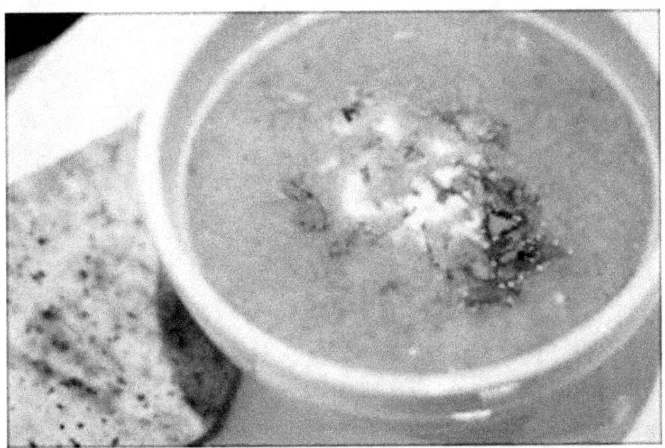

Chicken Noodle Soup

What's in it:

- 1 tbsp. lemon juice
- ¼ C. chopped parsley
- ¼ tsp. crushed celery seeds
- ½ tsp. sage
- ½ tsp. crushed rosemary
- ¾ tsp. thyme
- 1 C. water
- 6 C. chicken broth
- 3 tbsp. extra virgin olive oil
- 3-5 minced garlic cloves
- 4 chopped stalks celery
- 1 chopped onion
- 2 C. wide egg noodles
- Pepper and salt
- 2 bay leaves
- 5 peeled/chopped carrots
- 1 ½ pounds boneless skinless chicken breast

How it's made:

- Place chicken, garlic, celery, onion, and carrots to slow cooker.
- Then add bay leaves, rosemary, thyme water, broth, and olive oil, using pepper and salt to season.
- Set slow cooker to low to cook 6-7 hours.
- Take out the chicken and let rest 10 minutes. Cut into bite-sized pieces.
- Add parsley and egg noodles to cooker.

- Bump up the temp to high and cook 10 minutes till noodles become tender.
- Mix in lemon juice and toss diced chicken. Serve toasty with saltine crackers and a sprinkle of parmesan cheese is you like.

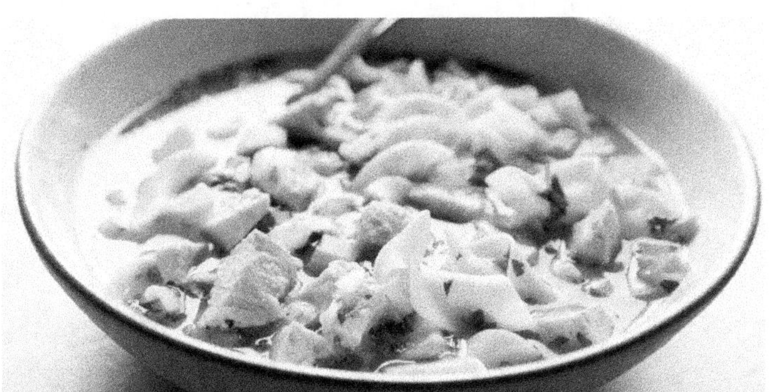

Dinner Recipes

Chicken Curry

What's in it:

- 1 sweet onion
- 4 C. sweet potatoes
- 2 crushed garlic cloves
- 2 tbsp. butter
- 1 C. water
- 2 15-ounce cans coconut milk
- 1 tsp. sugar
- 2 tsp. salt
- 1 tsp. turmeric
- ½ tsp. coriander
- 3 tbsp. mild curry powder
- 1 pound chicken breast

How it's made:

- Combine sugar, salt, coriander, turmeric, and curry powder together.
- Put chicken in the slow cooker and pour coconut milk and water over the top.
- Add garlic and butter to seasonings and stir well. Add onions and sweet potatoes to slow cooker along with seasoning mixture.
- Set slow cooker to low to cook 6-8 hours or Set slow cooker to high to cook 4-6 hours.
- During the last half an hour of cooking, take out chicken and shred. Then pour back in for remaining cooking time.
- Serve with rice!

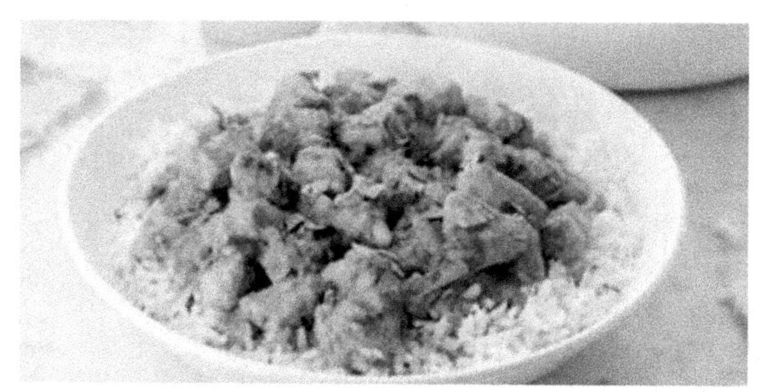

Easy Roast Beef

What's in it:

- 3 minced cloves garlic
- 1 ½ tsp. crushed red pepper flakes
- 2 tsp. basil
- 1 tsp. pepper
- 1 tsp. + 1 tbsp. olive oil
- 2 tbsp. salt
- 2 ½ pound boneless eye-round roast

How it's made:

- The day before you plan to cook roast, sprinkle salt over meat and wrap it in plastic wrap. Chill overnight.
- The next day, place roast in the slow cooker along with remaining ingredients.
- Set slow cooker to low to cook 8 hours till meat is tender.

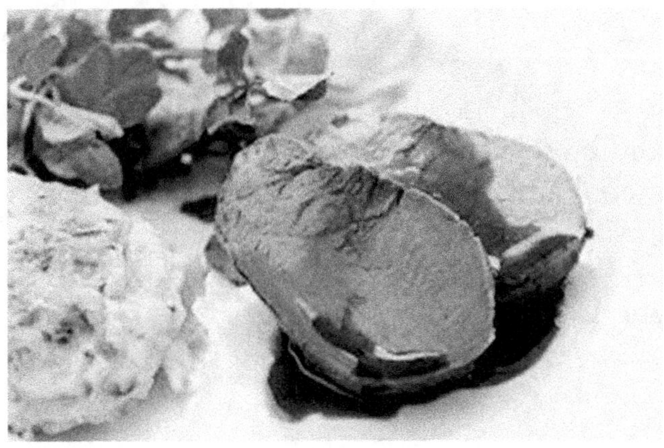

Pork Roast

What's in it:

- 2 tbsp. cold water
- 2 tbsp. cornstarch
- Pepper
- 1 tsp. garlic powder
- 1 tsp. salt
- 2 tsp. dry mustard
- 3 tbsp. red wine vinegar
- 1/3 C. soy sauce
- 1/3 C. honey
- 2 tbsp. olive oil
- Pork loin roast

How it's made:

- Grease your slow cooker.
- Warm up oil. Season roast with pepper and salt and brown sides in the pan. Place roast in slow cooker. Scrape bits from pan into cooker as well, lots of flavor in there!
- Mix pepper, garlic powder, salt, mustard, vinegar, soy sauce, and honey together. Pour over roast.
- Set slow cooker to low to cook 5-7 hours.
- Take out roast and place on serving platter.
- Pour cooking liquids into a pan, along with cornstarch and water. Cook until thickened. Serve with roast.

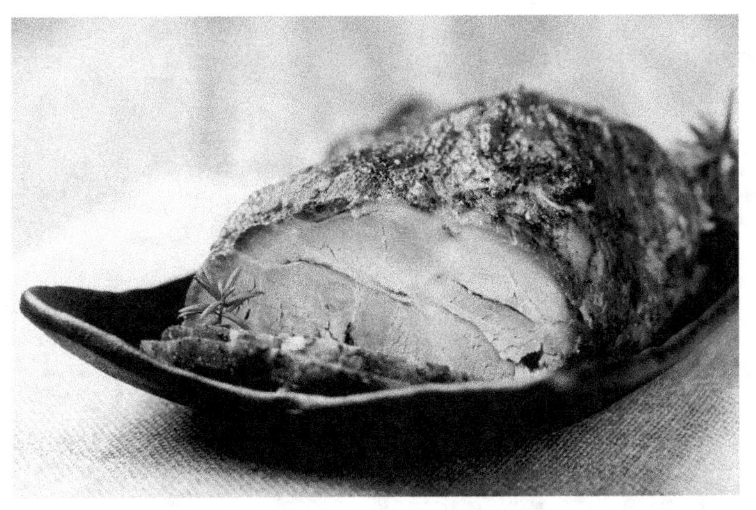

Onion Cream Pork Chops

What's in it:

- 1/8 tsp pepper
- ¼ tsp. salt
- ½ C. milk
- 1/3 C. dry white wine
- 3 tbsp. ranch dressing mix
- 10 ounce can cream of mushroom soup
- 1 cream of onion soup mix
- 4 center cut pork chops

How it's made:

- Season pork chops with pepper and salt and place into slow cooker.
- Mix wine, ranch dressing mix, milk, and soup mixes together. Pour over meat.
- Set slow cooker to low to cook 3-4 hours. Enjoy!

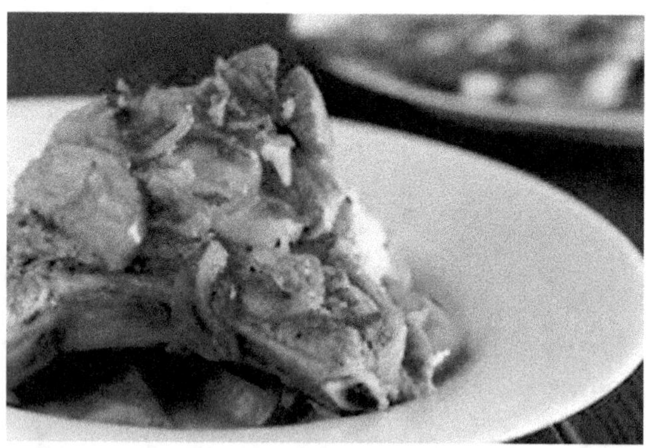

Lean Stuffed Peppers

What's in it:

- 1-2 tbsp. Italian seasoning
- 24-ounce jar pasta sauce
- 1 chopped onion
- 1 – 1 ½ pounds ground turkey
- 1 C. brown rice
- 4 green peppers, insides removed

How it's made:

- Mix together seasonings, onion, turkey and brown rice.
- Grease your slow cooker.
- Place peppers in slow cooker.
- Fill peppers with turkey mixture.
- Pour pasta sauce over stuffed peppers.
- Set slow cooker to low to cook 5-6 hours.

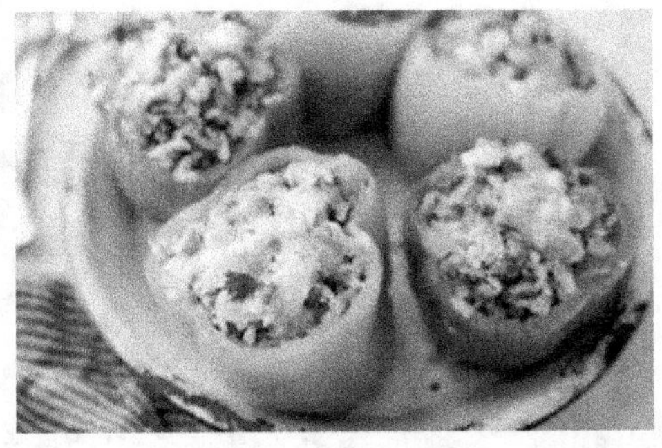

Brown Sugar Pineapple Ham

What's in it:

- 20 ounce can pineapple tidbits
- ½ C. pure maple syrup
- 3 C. brown sugar
- 1 fully-cooked spiral bone-in ham

How it's made:

- Spread 1 ½ cups brown sugar into the bottom of slow cooker.
- Put ham over sugar and pull apart slightly.
- Pour maple syrup between slices. Then drain pineapple and pour over ham, ensuring that some pieces end up between slices.
- Sprinkle remaining brown sugar over the top.
- Set slow cooker to high to cook 3 ½ - 4 hours or Set slow cooker to low to cook 6-7 hours.

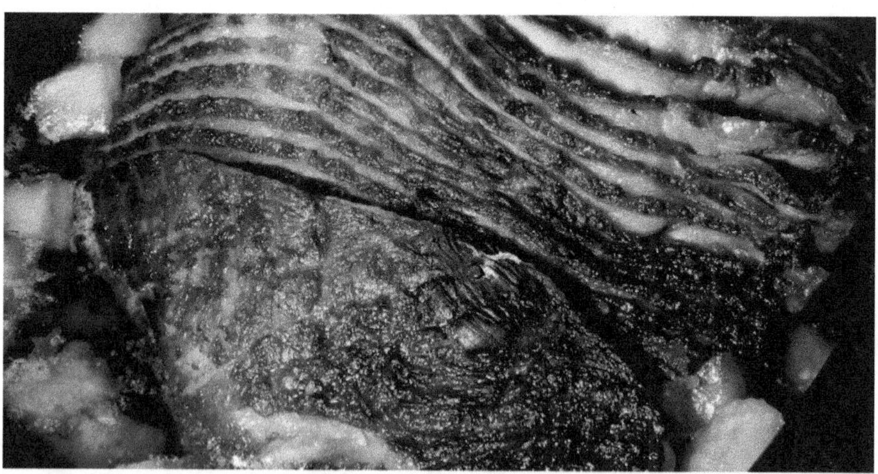

Crust-Less Pizza

What's in it:

- 2 C. shredded pizza blend cheese
- 14-ounce jar pizza sauce
- 2 C. shredded mozzarella cheese
- Garlic salt
- Pepper
- Dried minced onion
- 2 pounds ground beef
- Desired pizza toppings

How it's made:

- Cook ground beef and drain grease.
- Combine beef and mozzarella cheese together. Grease your slow cooker. Then spread out beef mixture into cooker.
- Pour in pizza sauce, spreading out evenly.
- Top with pizza cheese and desired toppings.
- Set slow cooker to low to cook 4 hours.

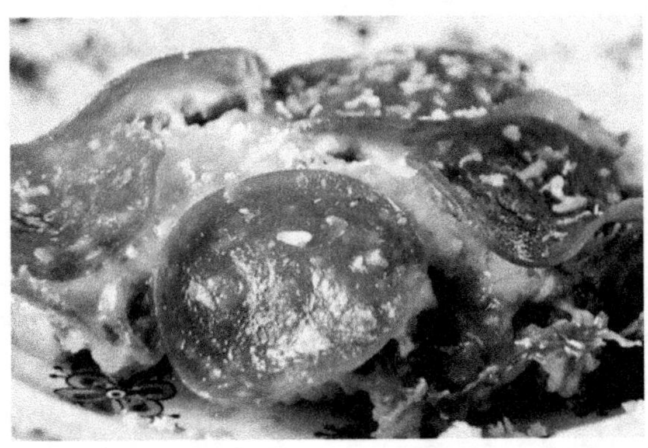

Orange Chicken and Broccoli

What's in it:

- 5 ½ C. broccoli florets
- 1 tsp. minced ginger
- 2 tsp. minced garlic
- 2 tbsp. sesame oil
- ¼ C. soy sauce
- ½ C. orange marmalade
- ¼ C. cornstarch
- Pepper and salt
- 4 boneless, skinless chicken breasts

How it's made:

- Grease your slow cooker.
- With pepper and salt, season chicken and put into a Ziploc baggie. Pour cornstarch into the bag and toss to coat meat. Place chicken in slow cooker.
- Whisk ginger, garlic, sesame oil, soy sauce, and orange marmalade together. Pour over chicken and stir to incorporate.
- Set slow cooker to low to cook 3-4 or set slow cooker to high to cook 1 ½ - 2 hours.
- During last 15 minutes, pour in broccoli.
- Serve with rice.

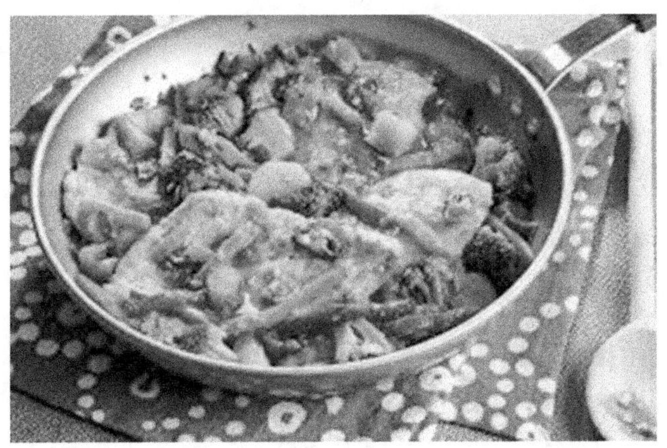

Roasted Red Pepper Chicken Chili

What's in it:

- 2 C. chicken broth
- 2 ½ tsp. salt
- 1 ½ tbsp. cumin
- 3 tbsp. chili powder
- 30 ounces red kidney beans
- 24 ounces roasted red peppers
- 2 tbsp. olive oil
- 4 minced cloves garlic
- 1 C. chopped celery
- 1 seeded/chopped red bell pepper
- 1 peeled/chopped onion
- 2 pounds boneless, skinless chicken breasts

How it's made:

- Warm up oil and sauté garlic, celery, peppers, and onions together 3-5 minutes till soft.
- Place sautéed veggies along with drained beans into slow cooker. Put chicken over top and season with salt, cumin, and chili powder.
- Pour roasted peppers in a blender and blend until smooth. Pour into the cooker.
- Set slow cooker to low to cook 6-8 hours or set slow cooker to high to cook 3-4 hours.
- Once the chicken is cooked, take out of cooker and shred. Place shredded meat back into the cooker and stir well to incorporate.

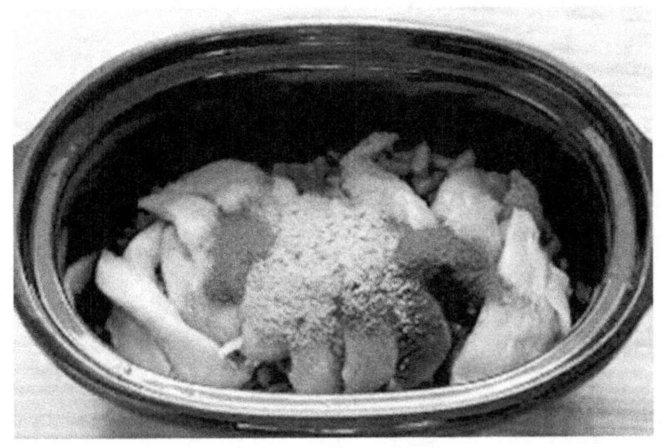

Apple Maple Pork Tenderloin

What's in it:

- 1 crushed garlic clove
- 1 tbsp. maple syrup
- 1 tbsp. balsamic vinegar
- 1 tbsp. Dijon mustard
- 2 tbsp. soy sauce
- 1 sliced apple of choice
- 2 C. baby potatoes
- 2 C. baby carrots
- Pork tenderloin

How it's made:

- Pour potatoes and carrots into slow cooker. Put pork tenderloin on top, followed by apple slices.
- Mix garlic, maple syrup, vinegar, mustard, and soy sauce together and pour over tenderloin.
- Set slow cooker to low to cook 6-8 hours.

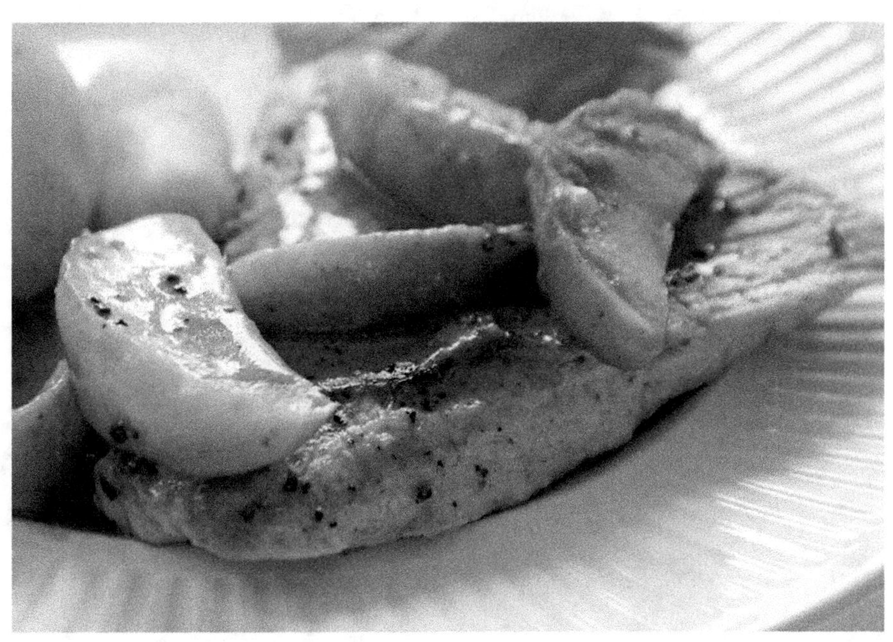

Dessert Recipes

Apple Crisp

What's in it:

Topping:

- 8 tbsp. melted unsalted butter
- ¼ tsp. salt
- 1 tsp. cinnamon
- ½ C. brown sugar
- ¾ C. rolled oats
- 1 ¼ C. all-purpose flour

Filling:

- 1 tbsp. lemon juice
- 1 tsp. cinnamon
- 2 tbsp. all-purpose flour
- 1/3 C. granulated sweetener of choice
- 6 apples of choice

How it's made:

- Mix salt, cinnamon, brown sugar, oats, and flour together. Stir in melted butter until mixture becomes crumbly. Set to the side.
- Grease slow cooker.
- Peel, core, and cut apples into 1-inch chunks.
- Add lemon juice, cinnamon, flour sugar, and apples to slow cooker. Spread out to an even layer.
- Sprinkle apples with crumble toppings.
- Pout paper towels over slow cooker. Cover and Set slow cooker to high to cook 1 ½ hours or Set slow cooker to low to cook 2 ½ - 3 hours.

- Take off paper towels. Cook uncovered 15 minutes till crispy.

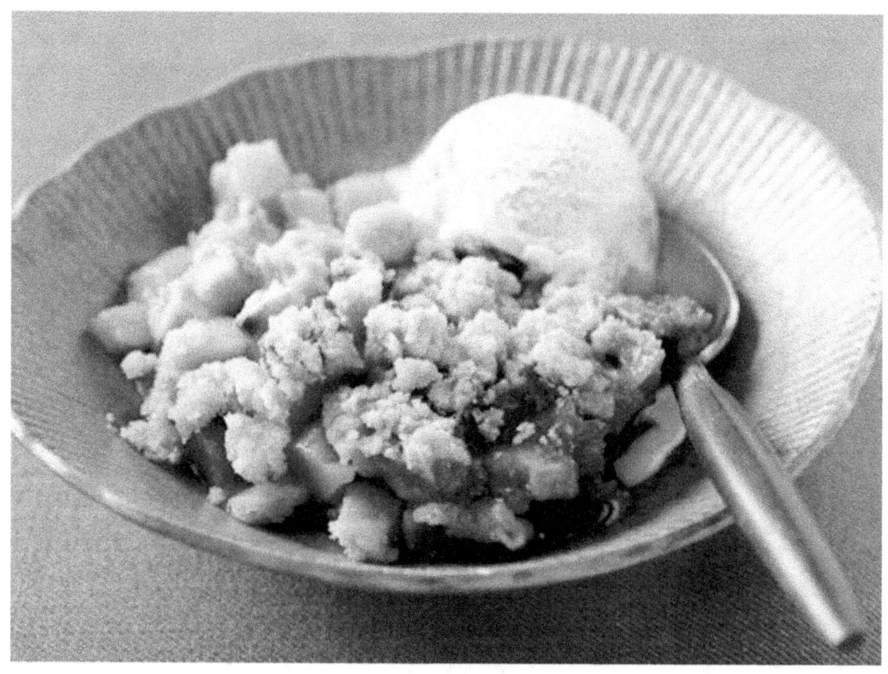

Cranberry Applesauce

What's in it:

- 12 ounces fresh cranberries
- 10 whole apples of choice (I personally like the taste of golden delicious apples with this recipe!)

How it's made:

- Peel, core, and chop apples. Pour into your slow cooker.
- Rinse cranberries and drain well. Pour into the slow cooker with apples.
- Set slow cooker to low to cook 4-6 hours till the mixture becomes saucy.
- Mix in sweetened of choice if you desire.
- Eat as is or blend in a blender for a smoother texture.

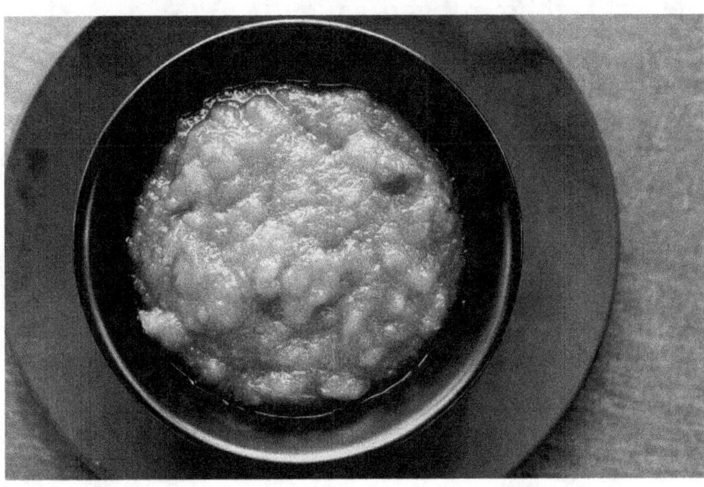

Fudgy Dark Chocolate Brownies

What's in it:

- ¾ C. pure maple syrup
- 6 tbsp. nonfat Greek yogurt
- 1 ½ tsp. vanilla extract
- 3 tbsp. unsalted butter
- 3 room temp eggs
- ½ tsp. salt
- ¼ tsp. baking powder
- 1 C. + 2 tbsp. unsweetened cocoa powder
- 1 C. + 2 tbsp. white whole wheat flour

How it's made:

- Grease your slow cooker.
- Whisk salt, baking powder, cocoa powder, cocoa powder, and flour together.
- Mix vanilla extract, eggs, and butter together. Mix in Greek yogurt, stirring till no lumps are visible. Then mix in maple syrup.
- Incorporate wet and dry mixtures together.
- Pour batter into slow cooker.
- Set slow cooker to low to cook 1 ½ - 2 hours.
- Allow to cool to room temp 4 hours to become fudgy.

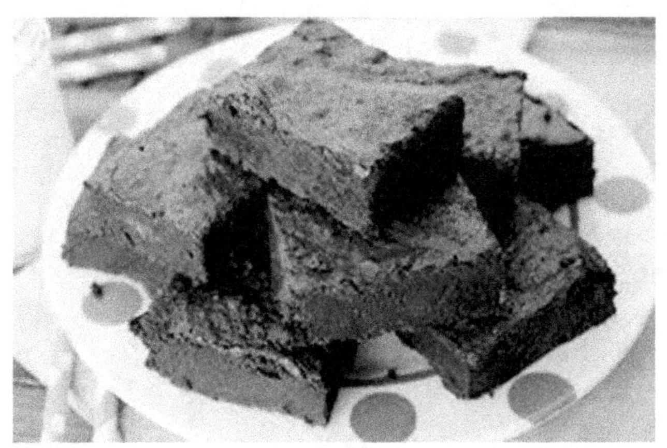

Poached Pears

What's in it:

- ¼ C. chopped walnuts
- 2 cinnamon sticks
- 1 C. apple juice
- 4 pears of choice

How it's made:

- Pour apple juice into slow cooker.
- Put pears on their sides within the juice, add cinnamon sticks.
- Set slow cooker to high to cook 1 hour or Set slow cooker to low to cook 2 hours.
- Open halfway through cooking and flip pears to other side.
- Place pears onto a plate after cooking.
- Put juice through the mesh into a pan. Add cinnamon sticks and bring the mixture up to boiling. Let boil 15 minutes.
- When the juice has reduced to a thin syrup, take off heat and mix in walnuts.
- Place pears on plate and spoon syrup and nuts. Enjoy!

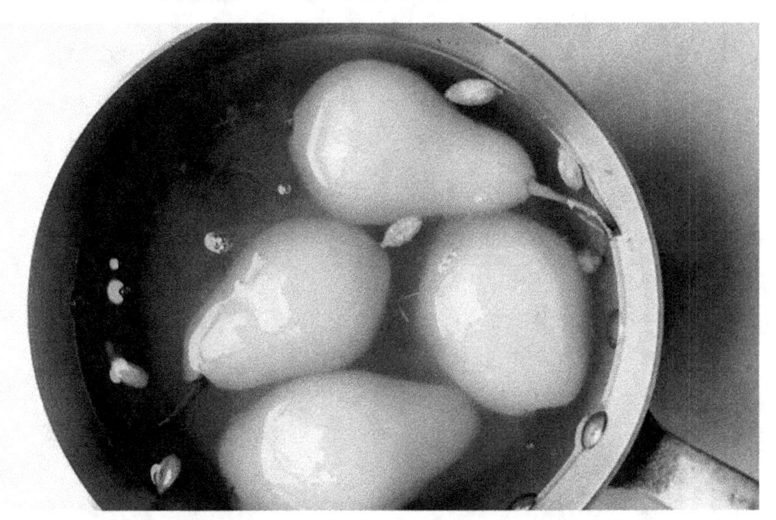

Arroz Con Leche

What's in it:

- 2 C. cold milk
- 3 C. water
- 1 C. long grain white rice
- 2/3 C. condensed milk
- ¼ tsp. vanilla extract
- ¼ tsp. cinnamon

How it's made:

- Pour in all recipe components minus the cold milk.
- Set slow cooker to low to cook 1 ½ hours till rice is tender.
- Turn off slow cooker and add milk. Mix well and let sit 15 minutes.
- Mix well before serving.

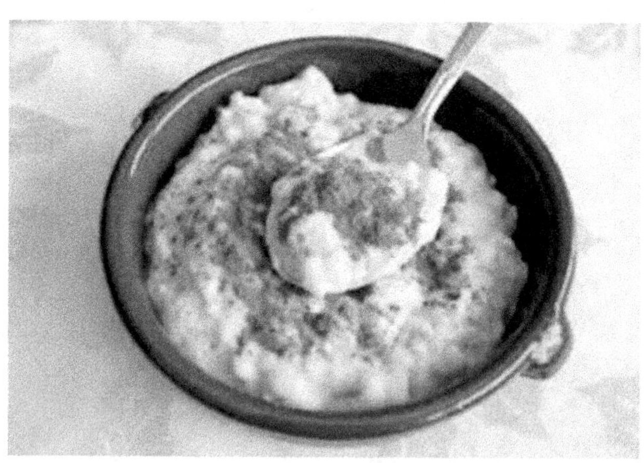

Blueberry Banana Bread

What's in it:

- 1 tsp. vanilla extract
- 1 tsp. cinnamon
- Pinch of salt
- 2 ripe bananas
- 2 eggs
- 4 tbsp. maple syrup
- ½ C. coconut oil
- ½ C. blueberries
- 1 C. self-rising flour

How it's made:

- Melt maple syrup and coconut oil together. Then add eggs, beating well. Stir in bananas.
- Mix vanilla, cinnamon, salt, and flour together and then mix with syrup mixture. Fold in blueberries.
- Grease your slow cooker. Place a cake pan in slow cooker. Pour batter into the pan.
- Set slow cooker to high to cook 1 ½ - 2 hours.
- Use a butter knife to pull out the cake. Cool, cut and serve!

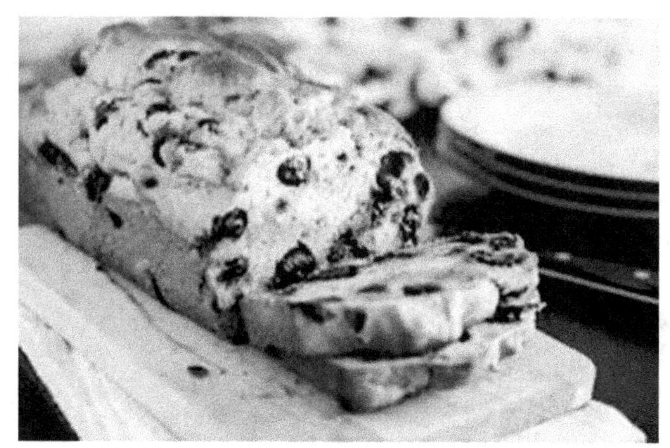

Pumpkin Spice Baked Apples

What's in it:

- 1/3 C. boiling water
- 4 apples
- 1 tsp. pumpkin spice
- 2 tbsp. sultanas
- 2 tbsp. walnuts
- 3 tbsp. cold butter
- 1/3 C. brown sugar

How it's made:

- To make the filling, cut butter into brown sugar. Chop walnuts and mix pumpkin spice and sultanas together.
- To prepare the apples, cut off the tops and core apple with the melon baller.
- Spoon filling into apples, packing it in.
- Place stuffed apples in slow cooker.
- Pour boiling water around apples. Set slow cooker to high to cook 2 ½ hours.
- Serve with cream and spoonful of cooking juices.

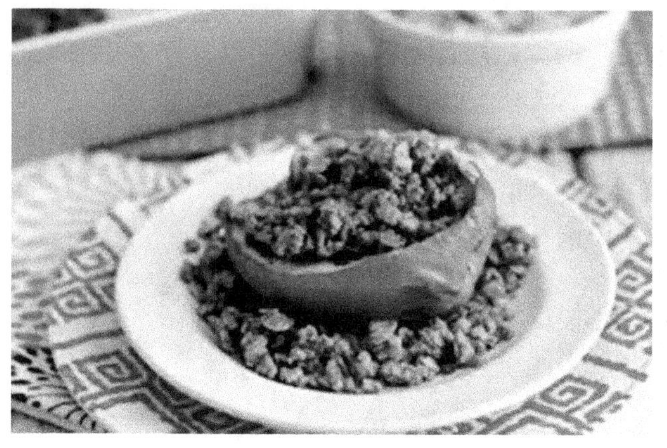

Orange Tapioca Pudding

What's in it:

- 3 oranges
- 1 tsp. vanilla extract
- ½ C. sugar
- ½ C. pearl tapioca
- 3 C. reduced-fat milk

How it's made:

- Grease your slow cooker.
- Add vanilla, sugar, tapioca, milk, and zest of 1 orange into slow cooker.
- Stir well to incorporate.
- Set slow cooker to low to cook 2 hours.
- Ensure oven is preheated to 400 degrees as tapioca cooks.
- Slice oranges into wedges and place skin side down onto the tray.
  Roast 20-25 minutes. Remove and let cool. Cut off orange flesh.
- Whisk orange flesh into slow cooker. Cook on low for another half an hour.
  Turn off the cooker and let sit 30 minutes to allow mixture to thicken.

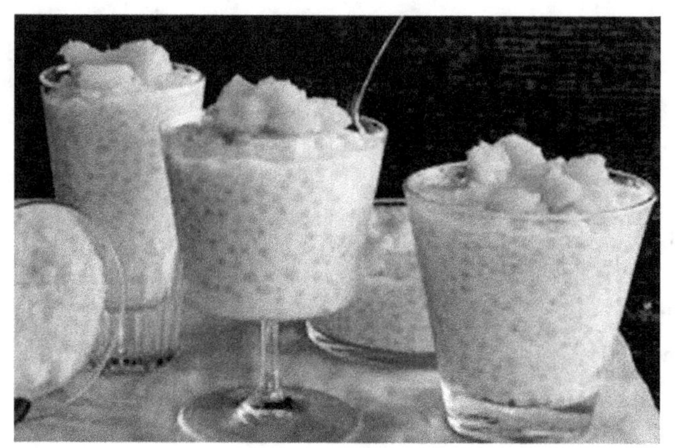

Chocolate Nut Clusters

What's in it:

- ¼ C. bittersweet chocolate
- 12 ounces semi-sweet chocolate
- 12 ounces jar salted/roasted peanuts
- 12 ounces shelled/toasted walnuts
- 12 ounces shelled/toasted pecans

How it's made:

- Pour all recipe components into your slow cooker.
- Set slow cooker to low to cook 1 hour till chocolate is melted.
- Stir mixture.
- Place spoonfuls of mixture onto wax paper. Allow to harden before putting them in a container or devouring them.

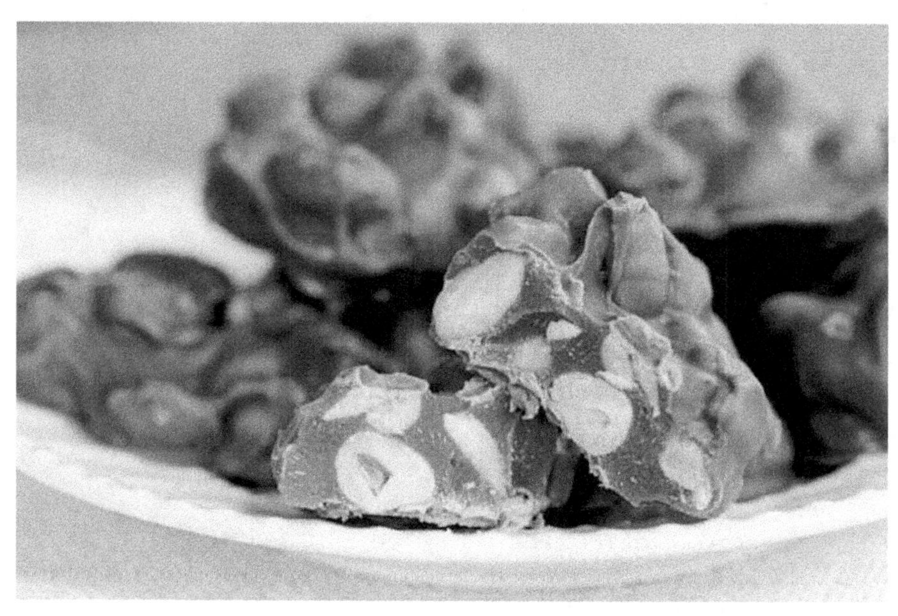

Slow Cooker Cinnamon Rolls

What's in it:

Dough:

- 2 – 2 ½ C. whole wheat flour
- 2 ¼ tsp. dry yeast
- ½ tsp. salt
- 2 tbsp. coconut sugar
- ½ tbsp. melted unsalted butter
- ¾ C. warm nonfat milk

Filling:

- ½ tbsp. melted unsalted butter
- 2 tsp. cinnamon
- 6 tbsp. coconut sugar

How it's made:

- With foil, line your slow cooker. Spray with non-stick spray.
- Mix salt, sugar, butter, and milk together. Sprinkle yeast over the top and allow 15 minutes for yeast to do its thing. Then mix in 1 ½ cups flour.
- Turn out dough into a floured surface, kneading 3-5 minutes. Let dough rest.
- To make the filling, stir all of filling components together till combined.
- Roll dough out into a rectangle. Sprinkle with cinnamon sugar. Roll and pinch to seal edges.
- Slice log into 12 pieces and place rolls into slow cooker.

- Set to bake on low 1 ½ hours till rolls are bubbly and firm.
- Allow to cool 10 minutes before carefully removing and devouring!

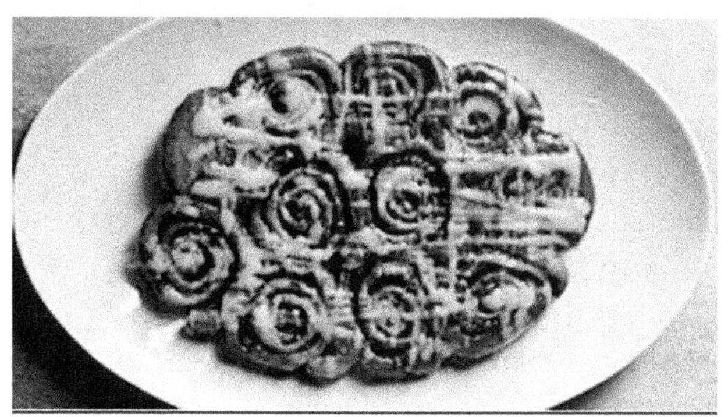

Drink Recipes

Kahlua Hot Cocoa

What's in it:

- 1 C. coffee flavored liquor
- 3 cinnamon sticks
- 1 C. semi-sweet chocolate chips
- 1 C. half and half
- 4 C. milk

How it's made:

- Mix all recipe components within a slow cooker, except coffee flavored liquor.
- Set slow cooker to high to cook for 2 hours, making sure to stir every 30 minutes.
- Once 2 hours is up, turn to warm and then stir in liquor.
- Serve hot!

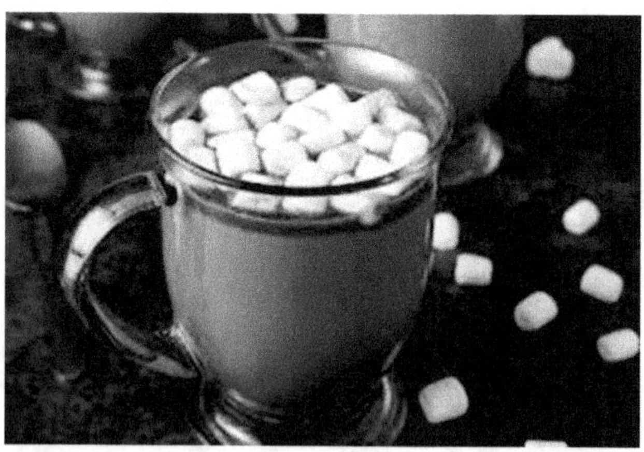

Caramel Hot Chocolate

What's in it:

- ½ tsp. vanilla extract
- 1/3 C. + 1 tbsp. caramel ice cream topping
- 2 C. milk chocolate chips
- 2 C. half and half
- 4 C. whole milk
- Whipped cream

How it's made:

- Pour vanilla extract, caramel cream topping, chocolate chips, half and half, and milk into your slow cooker.
- Set slow cooker to low to cook 2-3 hours till chocolate chips are melted. Make sure you stir the mixture every half an hour.
- Spoon mixture into mugs and top with whipped cream.

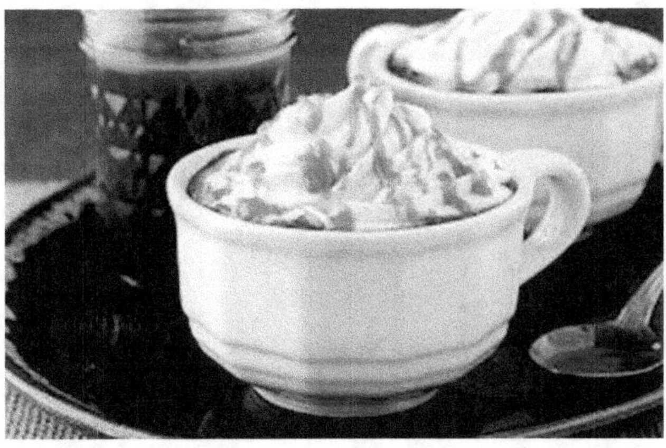

Caramel Apple Cider

What's in it:

- 1/3 C. caramel sauce
- 1/3 C. brown sugar
- 8 C. water
- ¼ tsp. allspice
- 1 whole clove
- ½ tsp. nutmeg
- 2 cinnamon sticks
- 1 orange
- 5 apples of choice

How it's made:

- Wash oranges and apples. Chop apples into quarters and place them into your slow cooker. Add water, allspice, clove, nutmeg, and cinnamon sticks.
- Set slow cooker to low to cook 6-8 hours or set to cook high 3-4 hours.
- With a fine mesh, strain contents into a pitcher.
- Mix in brown sugar and caramel sauce. Stir till dissolved.
- Serve toasty warm topped with whipped cream.

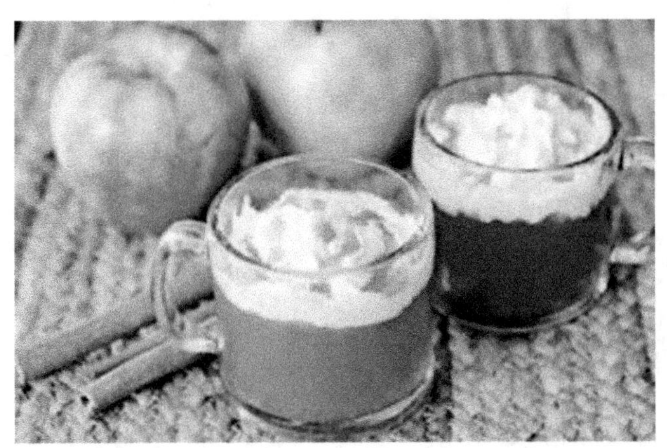

Wassail Bowl Punch

What's in it:

- 12 whole cloves
- 3 cinnamon sticks
- ¾ C. lemon juice
- 1 C. sugar
- 2 C. orange juice
- 4 C. unsweetened apple juice
- 4 C. cranberry juice
- 4 C. hot brewed coffee

How it's made:

- Mix coffee, cranberry juice, apple juice, orange juice, sugar, and lemon juice in slow cooker.
- Place cloves and cinnamon sticks in mesh cloth, tying it off and placing into juice liquid.
- Set slow cooker to high to cook 1 hour until mixture starts to boil.
- Trash spice bag and serve!

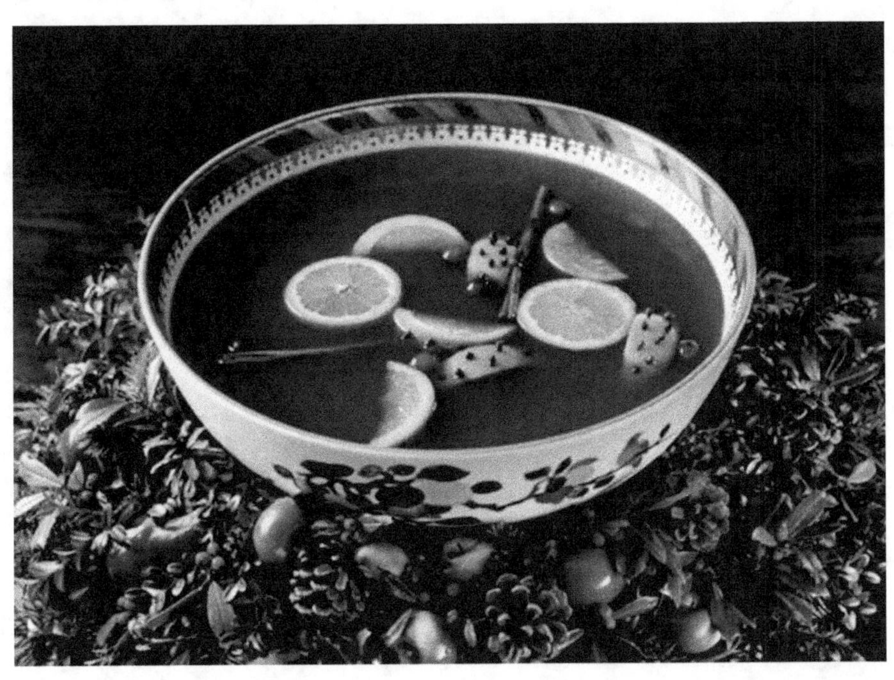

Viennese Coffee

What's in it:

- ¼ C. crème de cacao
- 1/3 C. heavy whipping cream
- 1 tsp. sugar
- 3 tbsp. chocolate syrup
- 3 C. strong brewed coffee

How it's made:

- Combine sugar, chocolate syrup, and coffee.
  Set slow cooker to low to cook 2 ½ hours.
- Mix in crème de cacao and heavy cream. Cook another
  half an hour till heated.
- Spoon into mugs. Serve with whipped cream and
  chocolate curls if you desire.

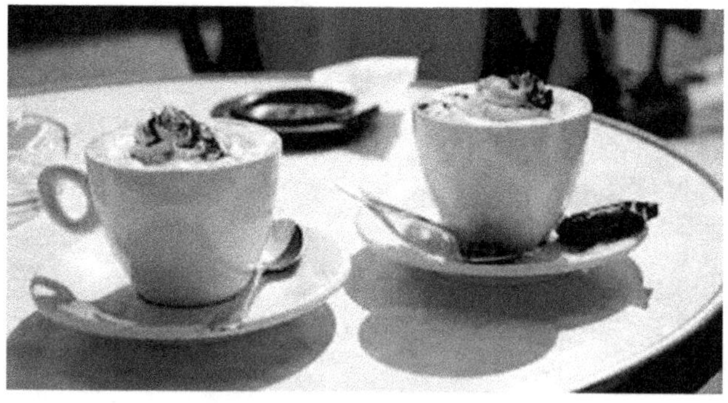

Hot Spiced Cherry Cider

What's in it:

- 2 packages cherry gelatin
- 2 cinnamon stick
- 1-gallon apple juice or apple cider

How it's made:

- Pour in cider along with cinnamon sticks into slow cooker.
- Set slow cooker to high to cook 3 hours.
- Mix in gelatin and cook 1 more hour.
- Remove cinnamon sticks and serve.

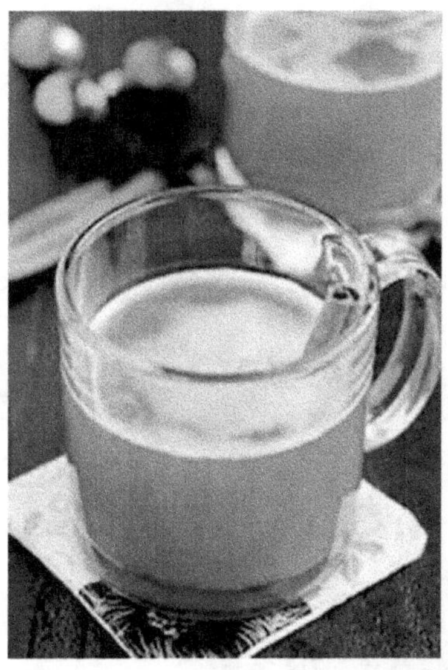

Spiced Coffee

What's in it:

- 1 ½ tsp. whole cloves
- 4 cinnamon sticks
- ½ tsp. anise extract
- ¼ C. chocolate syrup
- 1/3 C. sugar
- 8 C. brewed coffee

How it's made:

- Mix anise extract, chocolate syrup, sugar, and coffee together in slow cooker.
- Place cinnamon sticks and cloves in cheesecloth, tie it and place into the cooker.
- Set slow cooker to low to cook 2-3 minutes.
- Trash spice bag and serve with cinnamon sticks.

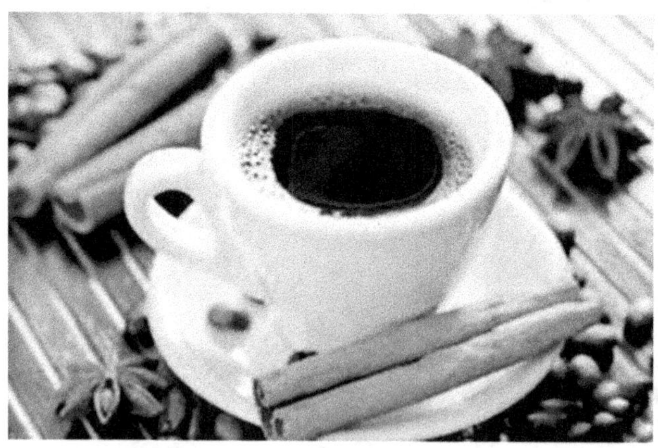

Hot Christmas Punch

What's in it:

- 1 package of Red Hot candies
- 1 quart unsweetened pineapple juice
- 1-quart orange juice
- 1 quart unsweetened apple juice
- 1 quart brewed tea

How it's made:

- Mix together all components within your slow cooker.
- Set slow cooker to low to cook 3-4 hours until candies melt. Make sure to stir on occasion. Serve!

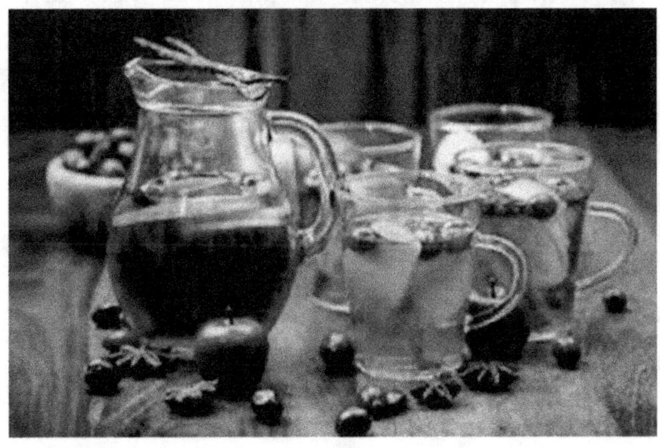

Chai Spiced Tea

What's in it:

- 14 ounce can sweetened condensed milk
- 8 black tea bags
- 3 ½ quarts water
- 3 whole peppercorns
- 15 cardamom pods
- 25 whole cloves
- 3 cinnamon sticks
- 15 slices ginger root

How it's made:

- Place ginger root, cinnamon sticks, cloves, cardamom pods, and peppercorns into a cheesecloth. Tie cheesecloth and place into the slow cooker with water.
- Set slow cooker to low to cook 8 hours. Throw away spice bag.
- Add black tea bags. Cook 3-5 minutes. Throw away bags and mix in milk.

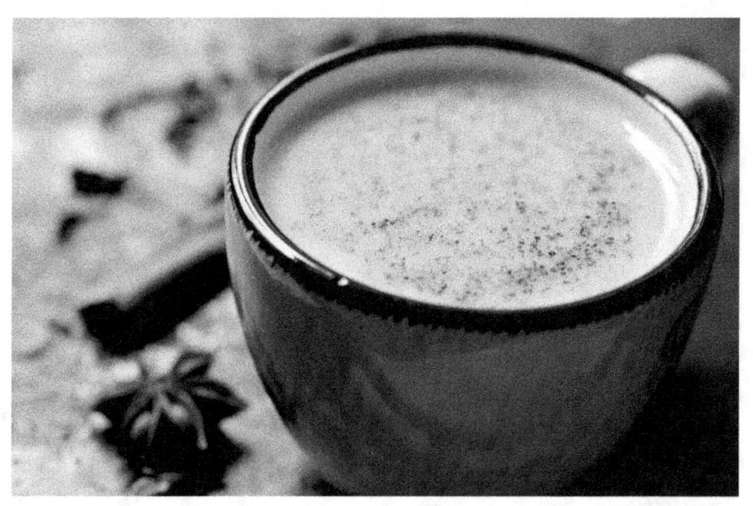

Peachy Spiced Cider

What's in it:

- 4 oranges slices
- ¼ tsp. nutmeg
- ¼ tsp. cinnamon
- ¼ - ½ ground ginger
- 2 C. apple juice
- 4 cans peach nectar

How it's made:

- Place peach nectar, apple juice, ginger, cinnamon, and nutmeg into slow cooker.
- Top with orange slices.
- Set slow cooker to low to cook 4-6 hours till everything is heated.
- Stir well before drinking. Enjoy!

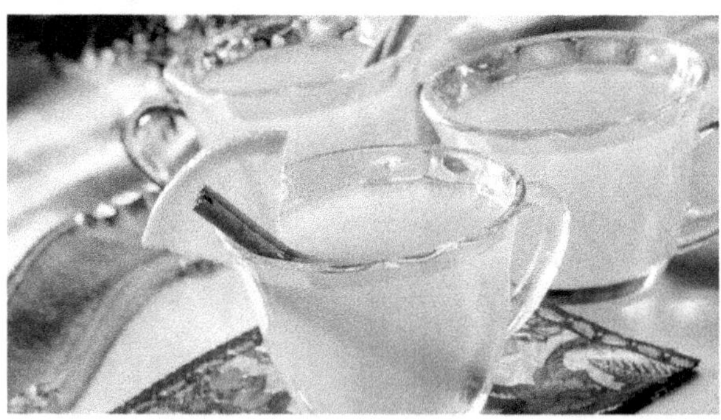

Conclusion

Congratulations on making it through to the end of *Slow Cooker Recipes*.

Now that you have had time to sift through the large variety of recipes tucked away within the pages of this cookbook, I have no doubt that you found a few recipes that made your mouth water and your stomach hungry for making new meals! I am sure many of these recipes will soon become family favorites! The best part is, you have this cookbook at your fingertips for life! So even if you only have the time to try one new recipe a week, you have many weeks of discovering new meals and learning more about your slow cooker to look forward to!

The slow cooker is an amazing kitchen gadget that many do not utilize to its full advantage! That is why I am so excited that you stumbled across this cookbook so that you can dust off your slow cooker and put it to good use! Or, if you don't already have one, now you have a great excuse to get yourself one of these convenient contraptions!

All you have to do now is pick a recipe, grab the supplies and see what the slow cooker can do for you!

I hope that you found this cookbook to be unique and unlike any other slow cooker books on the market. If you enjoyed it and found it useful in any way, please take a moment to leave some feedback on Amazon. Thank you so much and happy slow cooking!